dearlouisebook@gmail.com

@dearlouisebook

Dear Louise

Foreword

My mother died in November of 2002 after a relatively short and ultimately futile battle with cancer. I was twenty one years old and in the second year of a degree course at university in Sheffield. Now, in 2015, that event is over 13 years ago but is still the hardest time of my thirty-four years.

She, Penny, was a teacher at a state school, a bit of a hippy, and a strong feminist. She wasn't one for possessions so there were few things she let behind. The manuscript of the book you are about to read is a belonging most precious to me. It's seventy thousand odd of her own words, which I can read and which allow me to hear her voice in my head anytime I need to be close to her. Of course, she didn't write them to comfort her sons after her death – she wrote them to comfort herself during her life. As you will discover, my mother lost a daughter - my sister - as a baby, and that event shaped the rest of her life.

In the mid-nineties Penny tried to get this book published and wrote to a number of people. She had little success and twenty years ago as it was, there were no e-readers or easy routes to self-publishing. From the hand written notes on the printed transcript, it can be seen that she was still working on this book until around the turn of the millennium. Now in the digital age and because she always wanted these words to be read, I am releasing this book to the world.

Sam

"Perhaps one of the reasons my child chose me as her parent was because there was so much I needed to learn. "

Anne Wilson Schaef
"Meditations for Women Who Do Too Much."

Louise -

It's eighteen years since your conception. Nearly two decades to bring my book of you to the world. There are many reasons and some excuses for the delay but now my story of you is written and about to be read. And overall, the time lapse is no bad thing. Probably anyone who loses a baby is attracted to books of this sort – I remember I was. They describe the circumstances of birth and death, and their impact on the writer and those close to her, or, sometimes, him. It is incredibly helpful to know there is someone out there who has been through a similar thing and, at the very least, survived. Usually, though, such books are written nearer the event.

I have sometimes wondered, not so much how the writer felt after a much longer time lapse of, say, a decade, but how stable the restructuring of their life had been. Patterns of grief are themselves not dissimilar, but every personal world that grief destroys must be rebuilt, and a new identity created, piece by painful piece. This book is ostensibly about events of 1983 and 1984. It is much more about the impact of those events in creating the person I am now. In losing much of my life, I gained the strength to face, honestly, what remained.

There is another reason for the delay in completing this book, which has nothing to do with the demands of an over-committed life. For a very long time, I, ironically, conceived of this as a work of fiction - even when I started out. I spent a lot of the time planning a novel with you at its centre, exploring your impact on me. I wanted to create a new work of art from the experience of having you - to develop, and, I suppose, impose my own structure and pattern on those events. From the truth of all that you are I hoped to construct a new truth for an unknown audience.

Louise, I'm sorry. There may be material in what I've so far written that I can use, in this or other books, but my elegy for you should not be a fictional account. You are your own story, your own poem, your own dance. You are also, if I unfold this to you as it happened, the audience. I aim to be the instrument through which meanings are discovered and recorded, and I feel I have arrived at a stage in my life where I can be.

One main thing I have changed - the names of the characters, except for your brothers. Apart from the fact that those people and I may have shared intimate details of our lives, I cannot presume to speak for them. I have also altered place names where I considered it expedient. Occasionally, where I thought it might be helpful to elucidate the essential meaning of an event, I have changed the remembered pattern. This book is as definitive as I can make it.

Nothing can bring to me your living flesh or your touch: you will never hear the sea, feel its salt on your lips or see sunlight through a leaf. You will never know closeness to another human being. Your flesh is dead forever, as are the hopes and dreams I had for you. But language lives, as you live on in my universe, with all the love I had, waiting to give.

I could not give you life, Louise - this book is my gift to you.

Your mother,
Penny

Part One

Pendulum

1 Spring

I will bring you gold apples
and grapes made of rubies
that have shone in the eyes of
a prince in the breeze.

The Catholic Church has got it wrong. A pregnancy is, on average, nine calendar months plus six days, so Jesus would have been conceived about 19th March, rather than the 25th. For some reason, even in my times of lapsed Christianity, I remember Lady Day, and in 1983 I had reason to take more cognisance of it than usual. It was the date of my last period before your conception. On the day that, mythologically, the Word became incarnate, I experienced the last little death I would know before your birth. Two weeks later you arrived in my womb, ready to grow, develop and be nurtured. You were due on New Year's Eve. It seems an inevitable part of your destiny that you came to me at precisely the point where I'd decided, after all, that I didn't want another baby. I'm sorry.

I'm sorry- but at last, only for not wanting you more at that time - an apology that could be made to any baby, living or dead. For nearly a decade, crying sorry to you was loaded with self-blame: had I wanted you more, you would not have died. It's hard to articulate this thought because my conscious mind rarely did articulate it, yet my soul was sick with guilt. Slowly I let go, and in letting go I must accept that, if I am not to blame, even more of the story of your enigmatic life lies beyond my comprehension, just as much of my grief remains incomprehensible.

Recognising that dichotomy between mind and spirit, and what I had to try to do about it has, as I said, been a long process. Less lengthy, but just as significant on a daily basis, has been recognising the mind/spirit dichotomy I practised, especially in the year up to your birth. Feeling an intense dislocation between the reality I had and the one I wanted - I'll go into more details later - I constructed alternative realities in my head. It was the only way I could feel I had any control.

And then - - - you led me to a place beyond any possibility of control, a cave of darkness beyond understanding, where fantasy was a crumbled sword. I was in this world but not of it: I was wherever you were and wanted to stay there, with you, forever. Part of me still does. But I also knew that I owed it to my other children, to others who loved me, and most of all, to you, to continue living. If you cannot live, I must.

From somewhere came the strength to bear the unbearable, to know that the rest of my life would be a journey between your world and mine: sobbing, screaming, spilling out my insides into inchoate darkness in an attempt to reach you but, in between, bringing you into my world; showing you crocuses, the smell of hyacinths, the kiss of spring rain.

I had no choice in that cave but to surrender, to dissolve; to be reborn into a world where there was little to escape from because the worst had happened and it would inform the rest of my life. In breaking up my mind, you healed it.

2 Swing of the Pendulum

Bright cascading crystals
They dance in the sand dunes
On the beach with no footprints
To harpsichord tunes.

I'd decided, after all, that I didn't want another baby. Forgive me repeating that stark statement but it bisects time: a starting point to explore both past and future. I've told you of some of the impact your becoming flesh had on me. Now I need to explore the year before, when you were flesh less: I want to try and establish where you really came from. Having expected to have only two children, why had I then want a third? What did I hope to find?

The more obvious reading of that statement above emphasises a moment of choice: the image that comes to mind is a lump of marble containing- imprisoning - two mutually exclusive futures. Eventually I took the chisel of decision and released one - the one of no more children - sculpting bold, definitive, incontrovertible lines. The other future - you - would remain, forever, an unrealised possibility.

For much of that year it was like that - vague as a misty hill. But there's a less obvious reading that emphasises the length of time - that implies that the decision had been made before. And that is the more accurate one. For a year before you were conceived, my mind was a pendulum swinging relentlessly between two constructed worlds: tick - a world with you in it - tock - a world barren of you. Tick - I will have another baby. Tock - I will not have another baby. Each construction was, for me, equally valid, but felt qualitatively different: one had the etched definition of a stained glass window; the other, all the nuances of tone of pastels.

The images I invoked empty of you were the bold, primary, stained-glass ones. Here was the cleanness of completion: I had dripped lochia, blood and milk and now I could begin to reclaim my body and mind for myself. I could define myself from the outside because certain things were finished.

"These are my two sons."
"This is my husband."
"This is our house."
"This is our land."
"I am a writer."

Tick. Within an identity as strong, silky and seamless as the inside of an eggshell, my ocean mind would teem with shoals of words that I would trawl, breaking the sea's skin, or net as they darted within the diffuse sunlight surface. I would discover for each its precise purpose, guiding it to its fulfilment - and mine. Tick.

All the images that included you were hazy, mysterious, and potent with the promise of a different means of Becoming: a wing dipped into a rim of moonwater - the inexplicable significance of greeting you, of recognising you. Of holding you, moments old, in my arms, knowing, "so this is who you are!" And that, informing my completion.

"I have three children - two sons and a daughter."
"This is my husband."
"This is our house."
"This is our land."
"I am a writer."

Tock. The meaning of the last our sentences utterly changed by the first.
Tock.

Two constructed worlds, two possibilities - trying to create a diamond identity from within available options. It never occurred to me that, in different circumstances- for instance, if I'd been without a partner, or unable to have children - I would be attempting to define myself, and reach out towards the unchanging, from a different set of options, as closely proscribed by age and circumstance as these were. Tick Tock.

3 The Forest

A throne of white ivory
A gown of white lace
Lie still in the magic
Of the timeless place.

I assumed for a long time that my mind's year-long debate on whether or not to have a third child was purely about identity: of having to impose an external structure on myself because there was so little of an internal one. I think, primarily, it was that, and it's another forgiveness I need to ask: to look to your baby to help make you a definite person is heinous in the extreme. And of course it was your death, not your living, that taught me what I knew I preferred not to face; that my identity lay within me after all. I vaunted my spiritual values, yet spiritually, I was lazy and a coward: your dying was channels of light drenched water that licked my face and brought me to my awakening.

But it isn't just about the steely kernel of identity: it's about melding it with fluid gold; a sense of personal fulfilment forever changing the seemingly unchangeable; of knowing who you are because your being is full of experiences in which you are totally involved, where there was nothing left over. Why, at thirty-one, having married and had two children, did I find myself with little sense of self? At last, I'd done those things I'd grown up believing would fulfil my destiny - and they hadn't. They were highly significant experiences that had altered forever the flesh of my being without even approaching its seeds. So much inside remained unrealised.

For a long time I thought the fault lay within me; that I must, to paraphrase TS Eliot, have had the experience but missed the meaning. But however hard I tried, I found that love with a man was not the end of everything, and your brothers, while I loved them as much as any mother can love her children, were too separate from me, too different, for me to feel the promised fulfilment. I had expected that, in some way, I would reproduce myself, and from the day your grannie looked into your newborn eldest brother's cot and proclaimed that he looked just like his dad, I had felt like some kind of handmaid, having children that were nothing to do with me. Also, as both my parents were dead, all my legal ties were with males. But depression and worse lay behind facing that in fact, I had missed nothing: that there was no significant inner meaning to be had, beyond the experience itself.

Two paths diverged: in the forest of self-discovery I could reach my inner meaning with my sinuous mind, forging from the furnace of language, written patterns of perfect immutability. Or I could reach my inner meaning with flesh of my flesh, bone of my bone - my girl child.

You would be a gift of nature and I would nurture us according to what I believed. Like me you would be born at home; you would receive only breastmilk for the first six months. Like the adult me, as you grew up, you would wear dungarees and clothes of serviceable materials. You would learn survival skills and take your place in the world - your own person. Unlike me. But having become the child and adult I wanted to be, I would be free to let you go. Yes, it was naive, hopeless and an illusion. But such are the keepers of dreams.

But I also knew that if I could only bring myself to choose to have you, I was prepared to live with you not being everything I wanted. After all, the worst I could envisage was having another boy.

I was stranded in the forest, motionless in the curling mist of indecision, a knot of interrelated fears. I was very consciously, and deeply, afraid of living without choosing, the seeds of life itself withering inside me. I was much more afraid of those first steps, cutting me off forever from the other path.

I did a lot of research about what it was like to have three children. I sent off for information from the library, but other than a few statistics there was not a lot to be found out. There were no recorded interviews that I could find on the differences between having two children and having three: the answers are so obvious anyway that no-one had bothered to ask the question. I interviewed some people and wrote what they said into an article which was never accepted. I no longer have the article, but what I remember now is not its content but its subtext, which was a call for help and an attempt to make sense of this conflict.

In a series of mundane interviews, I asked parents how they coped with Three children, and received mundane, practical answers. Not only did I not know how to frame questions about how having a third child contributed to the meaning of one's life and the universe, especially if that child was a daughter - I did not even know that these were the questions I wanted to ask.

The months went past. Each first smudge of blood became another marker - a step along the way to becoming a writer, a woman in my own right, clean. Or it was an egg unmet, my body bleeding iron for you from its centre of breaking flesh.

4 Being and Doing

One hundred small children
they laugh at the white doves
that rest on their hands
with a touch of love.

Go, said the bird, for the leaves were full of children,
Hidden excitedly, containing laughter.
Go, go, go, said the bird; human kind
Cannot bear very much reality.

The pendulum swung, for most of that year before your conception, against the background of our house on the Lincolnshire Fens. We lived there for nearly four years, and both your older brothers were born at Pilgrim Hospital, Boston. Your dad had been offered a teaching job in the town, and with it the chance to rent a school house, from the Local Authority. The house was in a village called Stainton, about eight miles away. I gave up my own teaching job to go, knowing I was sacrificing my career, and my place in the world, but feeling that I no longer wanted to work within "the system." I can remember no other place to which I've moved with so much hope, yet left with so few regrets.

I've looked up a few diary entries from early 1979. How well I knew what I wanted - and how slenderly I knew my self.

Sunday 18th February
We are moving to Lincolnshire in April. In most ways I am very pleased: it will provide an opportunity for writing ... we will have a garden, and an orchard, and so will be able to provide a fair bit for ourselves. Also, the house is very cheap - £300 a year. I worry about the financial aspects, but with me having some time on my hands, we should be able to save money. In many ways it seems absolutely idyllic. I still don't like the idea of being economically dependent on my husband, but if I am going to write, that is a prerequisite - and I would rather write than anything else.

Sunday 25th February
On Thursday we went to Boston, and saw the house to which we will be moving. It needs a lot of work, but it will be worthwhile ..... There are many fruit trees, bearing Cox's Orange Pippins, pears and plums, and bushes of gooseberries and sloes. The vegetable garden is also in a reasonable state.

Wednesday 7th March
I am so looking forward to moving. I spend so much time thinking about Stainton, and living there, that spiritually I inhabit the house already. It only remains to shift our personal effects.

Monday 2nd April
My period is now three days late, so the chances are that I'm pregnant. I am pleased, but I'll have to do lots of reading on childbirth: I wake up in the night, worrying about it, and also the

enormity of the commitment. But I think that, at the moment, it's because I can afford these feelings: if it's confirmed, I'll be fine.

I can hardly believe that I stand so near the life I've wanted for so long ... we are moving to the country: I will have time ... to grow things ... to read, but above all, to write. And on top of that, I could be having a baby! Tonight, we worked out something of importance: that whereas, previously, I had relied on the day-to-day routine to keep - I suppose, my sanity - and had been scared of the void, the failure to relate, which lay behind it, I now no longer need it, and, in a sense, resent it because it is preventing me becoming what I want to become.

Being. Being was doing. Living in my future, my mind painting soft-toned images of fluid movement, easy sounds: crafting words - picking apples - making jam - planting potatoes - painting walls - cooking casseroles - breastfeeding a baby - playing with a toddler. No images of washing up, vacuuming floors, loading washing. Eternally unhurried, never stressed, headachy, or, most notably, tired. My slim fantasy body moved, usually in jeans and smock tops, without strain.

Being was doing, time a blue balloon expanding infinitely, my achievements curled along its inside edges. Or the images were somehow videos that could be run simultaneously, or a collection of photographs to be unfolded and viewed at the same time. Time conquered by being what I wanted to become.

I am less struck now by this naïveté than by the original misconception: these activities I saw as segments of an orange enclosing the silently unturning centre of my self. In fact they usually turned out to be sections of the peel, laid flat. Instead of touching the mystical, I walked on a two-dimensional shape, afraid to discover its edges or means of support - the opposite, I suppose of discovering the earth is round.

For a long time, I blamed Lincolnshire itself, choosing to forget that it provided, so uncompromisingly, the things I'd so arrogantly claimed I wanted: isolation, poverty, lack of status. If only we ... had a phone, if I could drive, if the village had a pub, a social centre ... I felt that I was slowly dissolving, spreading over the land, melting in the stark truth: nobody knows I am here.

The land itself came to haunt me: relentlessly flat, unfolded, nothing hidden from the searching, inescapable sky. Bitterly black, it yielded sweeps of barley and wheat and roundnesses of fruit, inside its quilted patterns of drained fields. And when I had one, and then two babies, the quilt was the gritty struggle to survive, that smothered all I thought I would become, when I arrived with such hope.

In the fantasies, I had glided effortlessly through time: now I fought to control time - my babies, my house, my garden no longer a focus for moments of being but as areas of competence. Time was rigid compartments of work and relaxation, like the sturdy ice-cream containers I later used for storing Lego.

Yet I also believed that babies should feed and sleep on demand, be changed when necessary, and later, that they use the potty when they needed it. So a tension was built in, not only between their life rhythms and my cubes of routines, but also between the mutually incompatible activities of child care and keeping a house clean and tidy. I deferred to your brothers' needs, and the mess they made, but my mind was a wire zinging with stress alert to snap to sudden shouting followed by remorseful crying- "I'm sorry. I'm sorry. Mummy loves you." Sometimes, I smacked them, and it was always because I had lost control - not once did I think they deserved it. This, I thought, is not it; this is not it at all.

And so I latched on to you, my love, or to my writing, to fold back the quilt so I could breathe my own life again, when all I did not know was that I had been - and still was - spiritually and emotionally unprepared for the life I had chosen. Ironically, I often latched on to both at the same time. Somehow, if I had you, the writing would be better because it would come from a more fulfilled person. At those times I could never acknowledge that it would simply be more of the same. Yet at other times, that was precisely what I did admit to myself. I longed only to be free of the tie of young children and could countenance nothing that would prolong this agony. And that was the pendulum.

Yet even this is not the whole truth. Just over a year after we moved to Lincolnshire, while your big brother Benjamin was still a small baby, your dad came home from work one day and announced that he was giving up teaching. He was unemployed for the rest of the time we lived in Lincolnshire - another two-and-a-half years. For most of that time, we shared the childcare and the housework. So for two days, he would do his Open University work while I did the domestic things, on a different two days, I would attempt to write while he did the domestic things, and in the middle of the week and at weekends we would meet as a family. The poverty was grinding, but for two days a week, I largely escaped from your brothers' demands, and, in a very small way, could cast myself as a writer with small children. And not all the articles I wrote at the time went the way of the one about having a third child: some did get published. Yet while the financial rewards were derisory, and we were completely dependent on the State, I had to continue trying to believe in the person I had constructed when we first arrived, even if the reality tried to undermine that belief at every turn. That person was a writer who was happily married, lived on a self-sufficient smallholding and now, she had three young children. She had to have a daughter because she had not become who she wanted to be through having sons. Yes, I pretended, because human kind cannot bear very much reality. To admit that we were penniless, with no chance of feeding ourselves with our produce, let alone start up any smallholding, and that I was probably in the grip of post-natal depression, would have led to a much more malignant perspective.

I nearly succumbed to that perspective suddenly, in the summer of 1982. Your dad went away for a week to OU summer school. Despite having a friend to stay for the first couple of nights, I was convinced that, while I was asleep, or suddenly in the day, I would have a heart attack and die. My mother had died alone in this way in June 1978, three weeks after my dad had had a massive heart attack which he had survived, for a few weeks at least, because she had been there to summon medical help. This manner of death came to haunt me progressively that summer, whenever I was alone, but particularly when I was alone with your brothers. They would watch this happen in front of them, and be unable to summon help, and be in danger, or they would be unable to wake me one morning. Your dad being at home for much of the time eased that tension, but it always hovered, like the wings of a sparrowhawk, in my mind. I was terrified of his leaving, and spent the entire week sweating, with convincing pains in my chest. The pains never really went until after I lost you - when, I suppose, I really had something to think about.

So when your dad was offered a job on the South Coast, we went: he, because he'd faced, after all, the prospect of never working again, and didn't like it: me, because I could no longer face the isolation, the brooding spread of land, the poverty. I don't think I ever fully realised that, to live cheaply, you need money in the first place to set it up.

Far from seeing any of this as a failure I didn't even regard it as an opportunity for self-evaluation: circumstances alone had defeated us. The system into which we were returning was, I felt, merely a means to an end- not something I needed to retain my sanity, to keep at bay the unknown fears whose hot breaths slavered in corners of my defenceless being. Never could I admit to being unfit for the life I had chosen: to do so, or to believe for one rounded raindrop second that there might be no way back, would be to truly die.

This is my first diary entry for 1983 - the year you were conceived and born.

Monday 3rd January

We are hoping to "use" Paul's employer at least as much as it "uses" us. If we can get money from it, we hope to get a house we can do up for ourselves, with land ... (we'd had, and done, that already) ... Life is full of possibilities: I hope it continues to be.

When I packed, at the start of 1983, I still took, in my head, a home in the country, a smallholding, status as a writer - and, from time to time, my daughter.

5 The Women's Group

On a hillside of velvet
The children they lay down
and make fun of the grown-ups
with their silly frowns.

When Benjamin was about nineteen months old, and Sam still quite a small baby, I started to take them to a toddler group in the next village. I could not have got there if your dad had not been around to give us a lift: sometimes he would stay - the only man there. Sometimes he would drop us off and collect us at the end.

I began to live for Tuesday mornings: for the reminders that there were other women "out there" doing the same as I was, even if they weren't living in constant fear of sudden death: having nights of interrupted sleep, washing and drying nappies, playing with very young offspring and picking up after them. It also lifted me because many of the women were already living a life parallel to what I still wanted to achieve, and I gained more optimism by being close to them, almost as if I thought my life would become like theirs through some kind of process of osmosis.

There was one woman I felt particularly attracted to. Her name was Jan Moore. Before motherhood - i.e. in a previous existence - she had been a nurse. She had woolly chestnut hair, and actually in general she looked like Anita Roddick. She wore dungarees or jeans with ornately printed smocks. Sometimes she and her daughter Becky, who was a few months younger than Benjamin, wore Clothkits clothes. Often, Jan also wore clogs.

Apart from the fact that she only had one child, Jan seemed to have everything I wanted. She could drive, she was thin, she kept animals. And she and her husband were doing up their own house and she was making things for it. Even her vibrant hair was a statement that she existed. She did not write - her talents lay in other directions. But other than that, while the magic still clung to me on Tuesday afternoons, I was Jan.

Although I liked a lot about Jan on a conscious level, even before I talked to her much I realised I had absorbed that she had very similar feminist views to my own. At one stage, she mentioned a women's group that she had been a member of for some time. I had never heard of it as it had arisen from a newsletter that did the rounds of people aiming towards real self-sufficiency. Women had met quite a few times, travelling considerable distances across the county in order to do so, but they had wanted to set up a group in our area, and no venue had been forthcoming. So to get us started, I offered to host a group meeting at our house. It was in the spring of 1982. Benjamin was two, Sam nearly one.

Apart from Jan, I knew - more vaguely - two other women in the group. The first was Tessa Hawthorne. She was a trained breastfeeding counsellor with the National Childbirth Trust, and although we were too geographically disparate to run a branch of the NCT, she had given me a lot of help and support that had enabled me to breastfeed Sam for eight months, although I had had to give up with Benjamin a lot earlier. I was probably one of her last clients, in fact. Her career as a freelance journalist was really beginning to take off, and she was writing so many articles for a parents' magazine that she was having to use two names. She had dark, rumpled hair and a dark blue rumpled smock. Tessa was softly-spoken, well-informed and slightly angular. She was married to an artist called Jeremy, had two daughters a few years older than Benjamin, and, like Jan, lived in a house she and her husband were doing up. For some reason, this project fascinated me.

A non-driver like me, she had been brought to the meeting by Olivia Barrett, the other woman I knew. The first time I met Olivia had been at an NCT Study Day that Tessa had organised in Boston, shortly before Sam was born. Most of our few subsequent meetings had been at Tessa's house, and, when Tessa came round after Sam's birth to see the new baby and offer advice, Olivia had brought her. Once met, Olivia was not easily forgotten. She was tall and large-boned, with slightly thyroid eyes which surveyed the world studiously from behind large glasses with emerald green frames. She was widely read and full of practical knowledge and with a love of doing things. She wore gorgeous bright clothes and, I was to discover subsequently, was very supportive. Yet I tended, although I tried not to, to find her somewhat intimidating.

The other non-driver in the room was Sylvia and she had been brought to the meeting by Sally, whom she had known for a long time. Sylvia Thackeray had eyes the colour of chocolate, which looked as if a light had been turned out behind them. She had long straight, pale brown hair cut with a severe fringe. Sylvia had thin red lips and spoke with a deadened Lancashire accent, as though her words were flames fighting not to be extinguished. She was doing some temporary work potato-planting for a local farmer, and she was still wearing her work clothes. Her younger child, Matty, was being minded by Sally while she worked. Her older child, Daniel, had started school. Sylvia also announced that she was on a diet, so she had eaten just the vegetables out of the family stew that evening. And yet her jeans hung loosely on her.

Sally Lawrence, in contrast, looked like a slice of sunlight. Her hair and skin were golden. She smiled easily and even her perfect teeth seemed confident. She was small, moving in a way that suggested she was totally at home in her body, that each bone knew and accepted its allocated covering of muscle and flesh. And although the sun loved her, I got the impression that all the seasons were there for Sally - that she would look different in each one, but essentially part of it, close to it, with that same understanding smile.

Finally, there was Lynne Marten. She had driven furthest, having come over from Boston, so she was the only one of us that had an urban existence, and therefore more direct access to amenities. Lynne's main feature was her silver-framed glasses which somehow suggested that she was about to say something devastatingly relevant, either cutting or hilarious, which, in fact, she often was. Her dark hair, fine like mine but wavier at the edges, did not suggest it, neither did the somewhat sensible clothes she wore: somehow it was all there in the glint of her glasses, and the intelligence centred in her small grey eyes.

That first evening, we began tentatively. We were spread around my front room on furniture unmatched by age as well as by design. The lilac light of an April evening slanted over planted fields, into the dusking room. The wallpaper was Laura Ashley, put up by the previous tenant. I kept this as the only childfree room in the house, and now, despite the open fire, it retained the greying chill of underuse.

While we chatted nervously, your dad came in, bearing a tray of mugs and with a note pinned to his dungarees: I am not listening. We smiled, and drank, hands clasped round smooth, warm pottery. We were underway.

We began to share - our sense of isolation, our guilt in unhappy childcare and our previously unspoken fears of how we might damage our children because of it. We discovered that we had all had mothers who, in one way or another, had exhibited bizarre behaviours: hawks hovering ready to tear at the throat of our own experience of motherhood, and still, at our experience of ourselves.

We also, that first night, brainstormed a list of what we wanted to discuss, and before each subsequent meeting, one of us prepared a paper - mothers and motherhood, childbirth practices, abortion, housework ,marriage, menstruation, body size, depression - these were some of the issues we discussed. Neither purely a theoretical group nor a support group, we were articulate enough to analyse our position, and caring enough to share how that made us feel. The personal *was* the political.

On Wednesday evenings, the relentless ferris wheel that was my life would halt deliciously, let me off into a summer breeze and allow me to connect, the black land now pitted with gems that were these women, vividly glinting, linked with gossamer in impossibly beautiful angles.

Looking back, I realise now how narrow we were in scope and background. White, professional, married women in our thirties, we were, until a childless woman joined us in November, also mothers who'd found ourselves displaced by motherhood and who wanted to reclaim our lost ground. We discussed issues of concern to us. And yet, we felt, somehow, that the group put us in touch, not only with each other and ourselves, but with all women - that what we said, and thought, and felt truly mattered. That seems arrogant now, but was never conceived as such. As for me - I have loved women differently ever since.

Yet over the months I came to realise that all these women were completed in a way I still could not be. In their different ways, they had emerged from the forest - they had chosen. They had made what I was coming to see as the Woman's Decision - how much creativity to allow through their bodies, how much through their other work.

I considered this one night, as your dad slept steadily beside me. Social attitudes could change, and he and I were jointly responsible for childcare, but etymology summarised the essence of procreation: to father a child - the action of a moment; to mother the same child - the act of a lifetime.

And the sound of their laughter
Is the sound of the green sea
As it washed round the foot of
The seashell tree

One late September evening, meeting again in my house, we talked about abortion. Three of our group had, at one time or another, had a pregnancy terminated. Lynne had asked to prepare the discussion paper. Having succumbed to family pressure at seventeen to abort her unplanned baby, she felt personally involved and yet distant enough from the event to be objective. Her grey eyes peered shortsightedly through her silver-framed glasses as she quietly read a paper that was cogent and well-argued, drawing on a variety of sources as well as her personal experience. Although the termination had happened over half her lifetime ago, she knew exactly how old her child would have been and still missed her. But what impressed me most of all was that Lynne blamed no-one. She accepted with dignity that those who had effectively made the decision for her had done what they thought was best. When she had finished, a thick silence touched us all.

Sally and Sylvia had previously said they wanted to take part in the discussion, although the event, for them, was much more recent. They had both had pregnancies terminated about a month before the group started. For Sally it had been an easy decision, and I noted her comments about having three children for my article:

"I know people who have three children, and it's much harder work than you think it will be, having one more. I had two healthy children already - one of each - and the life I wanted. I milk my goats, make cheeses, run a playgroup, spin and weave. James and I are enjoying doing up our house. I just couldn't spread myself between three children. There was a blob that had to be got rid of. It never became a baby to me."

The evening sun shone on Sally's hair, which was like a cloud of honey. It was the only vague thing about her.

Olivia spoke next. Olivia was pregnant with her third child, due in December. She talked about why she hadn't had an abortion, although she had seriously considered it, living in poverty in a rented house she thought should be condemned, with a husband she continually thought of leaving, and two young boys she already regarded as hooligans. Her eyes, behind those huge glasses, surveyed us, unblinking. She lisped, but spoke forcefully.

"I would defend to the death any woman's" - she looked round at us again - "any woman's right to abortion on demand. But after Rowan had ruptured my uterus they said I could only ever have one more baby, and from that moment on, I wanted it. I felt that there was a little someone out there, waiting to come to me. So in the end, I told John, we're having this baby no matter what."

After this, the steadiness of Sylvia's voice was more poignant than tears would have been.

"I'd defend a woman's right too. That's what made my operation safe and clean. Where I could kick myself is getting pregnant in the first place. I've never enjoyed sex. The baby was conceived out of carelessness. And as soon as I knew, I also knew I couldn't have it. You know, after each of the two boys' births, I was so depressed. And one lot of depression just seemed to run into another. I did seek help, and I went to the hospital once at Boston, but no-one ever seemed to consider how physically difficult it was for me to actually get anywhere. So I gave up and plodded on. Now Matty is nearly ready for school. There's no way I could start again. But for me the baby is still real. I'd be a few weeks more pregnant than Olivia. The fact that your mother's a nutter with bizarre behaviour patterns doesn't always seem a good reason for the death penalty."

Mellow light faded instantly from my Laura Ashley lounge. Now it seemed stark and cramped as a cell. Olivia went silently to Sylvia and put her arms round her.

So far, I have selected scenes from a moonlit pool of memory that relates to you, to try to understand your meaning. This next scene is culled from that moonlit pool more graphically than most.

It always took me a long time to get to sleep after a women's group meeting: that night, I hardly slept at all. I rose early the next morning, even before your brothers. I put on my pale blue quilted dressing gown (present from your granny) and went downstairs. With hands of glass I made some tea and took it into the garden.

There was a stab of autumn in the air, and birdsong, but nothing visible moved. The world was shrouded in cling film. I sat on bench under the apple trees, my slippered feet, darkening with a tide-mark of dew, surrounded by rotting fruit. Brown reindeer were etched on my mug. I pictured a unicorn, white, galloping steadily away, knowing I am watching. I see the full extent of my oozing cowardice, in the lion's throat of courage it could take to make the Woman's Decision: risking all for the chance of one more baby, or destroying a child if that's what it took to retain the steely sheath of personal integrity.

The hard knots of fear at my centre are untied. I look down. My mug is empty but its white inside is diffused: cannot focus. Tears of shame pierce my eyes then brim over, running incontinently down my cheeks to meet below my chin. I feel the cooling damp circling over the skin of my feet but do not move.

Eventually my fingers trace the pattern on the mug. The reindeer are framed by icy pine trees. I have to come out of the forest. I have not the courage of Olivia, Sylvia, Sally or Lynne but, in choosing, I don't need it. I wipe away the tears with the back of my hand and feel my face harden to a mask. Suddenly aware of the weight of fruit around me, I stretch out my hand towards an apple. I can almost touch it. If only I could have you that easily - but I cannot risk more of what I already have. There is no unicorn and there will be no baby.

Looking up at the resilient sky, I slowly realise that, though they may seem as small as ring boxes, I have made decisions, and that what has brought me here can take me on. Marriage - two children - this house - this land - my writing. I feel as though an invisible hand as drawn a boundary round my clammy feet, defining who I am. Here. Now. Always.

I get up from the bench, moving easily. Now a breeze bends, stroking the veined underside of an apple leaf. I stride purposefully into the kitchen, pour your dad a cup of tea, and greet your brothers joyfully when they awake.

The doves circle over
And land in the trees
Where parrots are talking
Their words with such ease

It is a raw Monday morning, early in November. Just after seven, our newly-installed phone starts ringing. I pick it up, register that it's Sylvia speaking, and comment on the time.

"Yes, I'm sorry, but then everyone with young children gets up early. It's just that John - Olivia's husband - has just rung with some news. You remember Olivia was bleeding?"

"Yes." I recall Olivia complaining over the past week about a steady trickle of blood that meant she had to wear a pad all the time.

"Well, because of her history, they did an emergency Caesarean last night, and so far, everything's fine. And you'll never guess - the baby's a girl. Isn't that unbelievable? Isn't it wonderful?"

Part of my mind registers that, for the first time I have been aware, Sylvia's words are themselves tongues tinged with new life. But for now I must shelve that knowledge, having also been punched in the guts by the most all-consuming jealousy I've ever known.

"Incredible. Fantastic." I stand outside myself, hearing the right sounds straining from my tightened throat. I had reasoned myself out of having another baby, but there is no place for reason here. My soul, stumbling in darkness, has suddenly seen a mirror, and trembles with the shock of recognition. And I feel guilty because Sylvia, who has so much more reason than me to feel negative about Olivia's baby, sounds genuinely pleased. Feeling mean-spirited and ashamed, I stumble on, trying to hide my feelings, hoping Sylvia will not notice. It was the first time, and I don't think I did it very well. After I lost you, I was to hear the same news, of friends, many times, always with pain, jealousy and an intense feeling of betrayal. But the acting, at least, got easier.

The following afternoon, your dad drove Sylvia, her younger son Matty - Daniel was at school - your brothers and me to Pilgrim Hospital, Boston, the vast, dominating, rectangular concrete building in which I had given birth for the second time only the previous year, to see Olivia. Except for the flowers that Olivia had received, and her striking emerald glasses, everything in the room was white - white with holiness, peace and love. Her face too was chalky with tiredness, but lines had been smoothed out, as from a sheet. She smiled continuously.

"Isn't it good?" she said. And I knew it was. As soon as I saw her, I felt part of her radiance, part of her total fulfilment. She was completely positive, unafraid. She had literally, put her life on the line, and she had won through. Olivia deserved this moment of triumph. I felt privileged to be sharing it with her, and I also felt that I should be ashamed of my feelings the previous morning, but sheer pleasure for her drove even this from me. We weren't able to admire baby Amber, though, who was in Special Care, with some problems. Apparently, she had inherited her father's pale gold hair. At that stage, the problems were not bothering Olivia unduly. Despite the interest in alternative medicine that she had recently begun to explore, she seemed to have total faith in the Health Service. She had also had similar experiences with Rowan, and all had come right in the end. We hugged when Sylvia and I left, and I felt truly blessed.

Sylvia and I, squeezed in the car on the way home, could talk of nothing but Olivia - how beautiful she seemed, how wonderful the baby was going to be - we even began to speculate that John would probably get his act together now and make Olivia's life easier. We felt that Olivia had given the whole women's group the gift of a girl child - a new female for our future. However, I noticed that your dad remained steadfastly silent throughout the journey, and I wonder now if that's what prompted Sylvia to observe, practically:

"Well, I suppose we can't really tell how things are going to be until all the euphoria's died down," and after that, we were all silent, even the children.

Slices of pale light fingered the naked embers of fields, reluctantly withdrawing their weakening support against accumulating cold and dark. Sylvia called in for coffee, as Sally had agreed to collect Daniel when she picked up Lucy, her own school-age child. Sylvia and I sat in my back room. the fire blazing, watching the children play with Benjamin's "Shufflies." These were little plastic people with fixed legs who, having some kind of see-saw mechanism attached to the soles of their feet, "shuffled" up and down their plastic castle, amusingly enough, we hoped, for the children not to disturb us while we attempted to have an adult conversation.

We talked again of Olivia, but now, away from the hospital, in more muted tones, and though our spirits were touched with the same flames, there was not the same unity as we had felt at the hospital. With distance for reflection, we were experiencing more of the impact that Amber was to have on our separate lives.

Sylvia was thrilled for Olivia, but now, somewhat sadly apart - Olivia's decision could never be right for her, and she had had to go to desperate lengths because of it. I still loved and respected Sylvia for her courage, which had informed my unicorn moment in the garden, and wished I could be as steadfast with my attempts at decisions. I respected her even more when, during our conversation, it emerged how much of her personal burden Sylvia was being called on to shoulder alone: when she had tentatively mentioned to Harry, her husband, that their own baby would have been due at this time, she heard only the response, "Don't go on about it," and he had left the room.

I had distance of a sort now, from Olivia, having seen her and discovered that, in having Amber, she had had only her own baby and taken nothing from me, but I had vicariously sipped at the well of mothering a daughter and burned with unquenched thirst. I felt that I could say nothing of this to Sylvia, who regarded herself as having destroyed her own child, but when we gave each other a big hug as she left, I did ask her to call any time she wanted to talk. Olivia was, in a unifying way, with us again.

It was towards the end of the same evening that I articulated the idea of another baby to your dad. I could not remember a time, since Sam was a young baby, when I had not thought about you, even if I'd so often rejected the idea, that I had forgotten what a shock it would be to him. We sat in the back room, watching the fire die. We had been going to get ready for bed when I began the conversation, and no lights were on.

"P., you know we can't afford another child. And there isn't room in this house. The two boys are brilliant together - all you'd do is spoil that. The world is stretched enough anyway, to feed the people already in it."

"You know that politically, it's a question of resource distribution, rather than sheer numbers," I replied curtly, trying to give the impression that I knew some facts and wasn't acting purely on an emotional level.

"Besides which," he went on, "what about your writing? You're always going on about it, and how frustrating it is when you can't do it. Another baby would delay it for years."

"Yes, but"… the words forced themselves out - "what if I get to the other end of my life and realise… that there… would have been time?" The question hung in the dark spaces of the room, unanswered. "It's all euphoric now," he told me, translating Sylvia's practical words into a comfortless parody; "but you won't be so keen once this has died down. Olivia will go back to moaning about John, the children - and she'll have one more - the mess, collecting firewood from the sea wall, the old Raeburn and her primitive existence generally. After a while, you'll realise it's not what you really want." He stood up, kissed the top of my head and went to bed.

In the fire, a couple of coals slipped with a whisper. I poked it, feeling for warmth, but its heart was gone, and my legs shivered. I loved, and was sharing my only life with, a man who knew not only what he wanted but what he thought I wanted too.

And yet he based what he had said around the events of the past two days. How could he know this was the culmination of so much searching? We had given each other children, work, kindness; we shared our bodies, a bed - we literally slept together. Yet my head, on a pillow, could be inches apart from his and for some time now, a large part of what was going on inside it had been unknown to him. I found this thought as empty as my womb was going to remain. I put the poker down and wrapped my arms around myself. The next period would be more than a loss of blood. It would be a loss of hope. Silently, I wept the first of many tears for you, Louise - my lost daughter.

8 Joshua

As an observer of my behaviour, your dad would have felt vindicated in his opinion. He would have noticed a time in which things resumed an even course, in which I rarely - if ever - alluded to the idea of another baby, and in which I became less tense. But this still had more to do with words that remained unspoken, and continuing what I had learnt at the hospital.

The euphoria surrounding Amber's birth did die down, more quickly than anyone had anticipated, because, after a few days, the baby became seriously ill with a blood disorder. One of the nurses spotted something badly wrong and the baby was given treatment in the nick of time. Subsequently she was fine, but it was a more muted joy brimming with gratitude and relief that replaced our initial high, once we knew all was well. Yet we also knew that this feeling, unlike that intensity, was immutable, even if it was her survival rather than her birth - more than her femaleness - that would forever make her life special.

Then, as I got to hold, talk to and to know baby Amber, for who she was rather than for who I had imagined she might be, I knew more certainly that she was a person in her own right who, like her mother, had enriched rather than diminished me.

Yet even as I let my jealousy go, without a core to my life, I found myself back among forgotten fantasies. When I took myself off to write, I was Tessa, except that her work was guaranteed an audience, and she was making something resembling a living from it. At other times I was Olivia, substituting writing for spinning and weaving. I had three children - it was simply that my daughter hadn't arrived yet.

Yet I could just as convincingly be Sylvia, Sally or Jan. If I was Sylvia or Sally, I would regard my family project as fulfilled. Again as Sally, or Jan, I fantasised about properly creating the self-sufficient life that your dad and I had chosen, including doing up the house. When I was Sylvia I fought to retain order, and your dad got nagged to keep everything clean and tidy and to put things away in neatly labelled ice-cream containers. I even considered dyeing my hair when Jan had a brief flirtation with an unenviable shade of green. Sometimes I could be other women, but I was these most consistently, and I was Tessa and Olivia the most. Yet I moved within the characters of these women without strain: yes, I was back in the forest, but, perhaps because Amber's birth and successful fight for life had made all things seem possible, or perhaps because we were moving soon, there were no deadlines to meet, no choices to be made, no pressure to choose one person to be that would exclude all others. I moved in time, but time was not a limitation.

There were still moments that could stab me, though. One night, at a women's group meeting, when Olivia was changing the baby's nappy, she looked at Amber's genital area, and commented,

"It's all so neat... so easy to put a nappy on. You don't have all this... stuff... waving around, that you have to try and tuck in." As she talked, she gesticulated graphically. All of us there that night had mothered sons, and we laughed, having encountered the same problem.

But what she said reminded me that babies are not just babies, that gender matters. Even to feminists. Especially to feminists. Feminists who want daughters because sons are politically unacceptable. And to this feminist, so rooted in her own gender that she still felt she hadn't reproduced, in having her sons - that somehow, they had been loaned to her.

It also struck me as ironic that, in celebrating the baby's genital neatness, and, by extension, that quality in our own bodies, we actually drew attention to something we chose not to regard as either biologically-determined or gender-specific - at least where our own children were concerned. Our own experiences had shown us precisely how socially filtered "neatness" was.

One evening, before the baby was born, Olivia had sat, splendid in a scarlet maternity dress. At first, we had laughed with her as she recounted how John dropped his dirty washing at the side of the washing basket rather than lifting the lid and putting it in. Then she'd added, soberly, "I've ranted and raved. I've even tried to leave him. I don't want to leave him. But I can think of nothing I can do to make him change. I am coming to the view that I will have to accept that."

The men of our generation had been pampered by mothers who did everything for them, and who berated daughters-in-law who failed to continue where they had left off. (Several years later, another friend's mother-in-law told her, "I don't know why you bothered getting married at all!" because, among other things, this friend didn't make her husband's sandwiches.) We could only do so much to change the habits of a lifetime if a man chose not to take responsibility for his own mess. But with our *own* children, we did have hope of making each child autonomous and self-responsible. We had agreed with Olivia, though, that girls were biologically neater than boys. Did we subconsciously extend that analogy? And if so, what hope was there for genuine change?

We were falling apart. Sally no longer needed the meetings - if she ever had - and went on milking her goats and making her cheeses without us. Jan's attendance was increasingly infrequent. Tessa was now doing high-powered writing, travelling to London a lot of the time, and generally moving outside our orbit. Olivia had applied for a Winston Churchill Scholarship that would enable her to study wools and their processing in New Zealand the following year. She planned to take the baby with her. I was headed for the South Coast. Sylvia was subject to periodic bouts of depression coinciding with the onset of winter.

To the excitement of all of us, she had recently taken a short-term contract teaching at a secondary school in Horncastle. I really thought that it would help us if one of us had a foothold again in the world "out there." But she hated it. The staff were unsupportive and the kids were riotous - rather as your dad had found in his teaching stint in Boston. I was so disappointed when she gave up that I remember curtly remarking,

"That bit of liberation didn't last long then, did it?" It was hardly the most supportive thing I could have said, but I just hadn't wanted to admit how complex the whole question of choice for women was, or that there were things women could do which were about as bad as childcare. Now, Sylvia didn't want to get up in the mornings and very little seemed to matter to her. I found it hard to accept that I couldn't reach her.

The only bright light on our horizon was a new member of our group. She had dark hair, wiry like Tessa's and eyes as dark as Sylvia's but rounder and kindled with enthusiasm. She wore playful clothes like stripy dungarees which suited her frame, accurately described by Olivia as *gamine*. Attractive, talkative and intelligent, Anna Saunders' twenty-year marriage had finally faded away, like a rainbow from a watery sky, and she was painfully starting to rebuild her life. Her priority was to find out who she was as a woman in her own right, rather than someone's wife.

Childless - not of her own choosing - in paid employment and with her own transport, Anna was in many ways atypical of the group, but the perceptive Olivia, whom she had met through a mutual friend, recognised at once the support that could be offered. It was precisely those qualities that we needed to be reminded that there was any kind of life that did not involve a permanent interaction with young children. Anna travelled to Peterborough and Norwich, joined other thriving women's groups, gave us access to books and ideas we had not previously encountered, and opened up new avenues for debate. It was Anna who introduced Sylvia to the immensely - for her - helpful "The Women's Room," and another book which began with the premise, "If a man wants to make love and you don't, it's his problem, not yours." Sylvia seemed to find this affirmatory, if sad. Anna was the proverbial breath of fresh air, and if the group was to survive its present fracturing, Anna would be the reason. It is now mid-December, and probably the last meeting at my house. We don't have an agenda, having intended this meeting as a social evening rather than a consciousness-raising exercise. But no-one can summon up much enthusiasm and the meeting finishes early. Anna gives Sylvia a lift home to her isolated semi; Lynne heads off for the humming throb of Boston. Amber sleeps while Olivia continues to knit for her the black Fair-Isle jumper - with matching hat - that she has been working on all evening. Olivia seems - understandably - to be in no mood to go home, and I make more tea. We are in the back room tonight. The light, beyond my trendy purple curtains - they had belonged to my mum - makes a small pool in the intense country darkness of the garden. I build up the fire and we sit either side of it, watching the flames. Hot drinks in our hands, we feel heartened, despite our concern for our friends. In silence we watch the flames for a few minutes, then, from what seems like a long distance, I hear Olivia say,

"I saw Helen Jones in town yesterday. She sends her love." I turn reluctantly to face Olivia, trying to focus my thoughts. Behind the large glasses her slightly convex eyes have a faraway look.

I quickly assemble Helen's image in my mind. I am not supposed to think this sort of thing anymore, but if there's anyone I would like to look like, it's Helen Jones. Facially she resembles Mia Farrow but she's less gaunt, less translucent. She has an average amount of flesh on an average skeleton. If I've wanted anything to do with my looks since teenage years it's to be attractive yet not different. And this is Helen. I realise that my hand has made an unconscious gesture towards my head, feeling for fairish curls.

"Thanks. How is she?"

"Fine, all things considered. Isaac seems to be a bit more settled now."

"Good."

I've only met Helen a few times but I feel I know her quite well because she knows most of the other women in the group, and usually, there is some reason why she is currently a topic of conversation. Helen would actively support the women's movement but for everything that gets dumped on her. She always seems to be the victim of a crisis not of her own making. She has been physically abused in two relationships that I know of, and her home was repossessed when her partner failed to maintain mortgage repayments. In the latest crisis, her four-year-old has been banned from his fifth playgroup for attacking other children. From being two, Isaac has steadily become more violent and there seems little that Helen - or anyone else - can do to stop him. Helen also has a daughter - Naomi - who is a few months old, and apart from the ordinary pressures of a breastfed, non-sleeping baby, she has to remain alert so that her daughter is not attacked by her son.

"You know," Olivia concludes, "she has known pain that we cannot even begin to comprehend." There is still the same faraway look in her eyes.

I say nothing, but inwardly I feel a bit indignant. Okay, so Helen's had a bad time, but then what about all our other friends? Then I realise that Olivia isn't alluding to any of Helen's much-aired problems, traumatic as they are. She is remembering that, a couple of years before, Helen lost a baby. Twelve weeks too early she went into labour and gave birth to baby Joshua. He lived for only a few hours. Helen is the only person I know who's lost a baby. Even so, I can't believe that this is substantially different from the other crises that Helen faces.

Olivia clearly thinks that it is, and I also feel patronised in some way. I want to point out what she already knows, apart from the collective problems of the women's group. I have had my own share of personal tragedy, my parents dying so suddenly in 1978. With your dad's support I came through - eventually - and initially, our move to this house helped. Olivia has made her statement and I am in no position to refute it, but I resent what seems to be a demotion in the league table of pain. I can conceive of suffering only in quantitative terms. I realise Helen must have suffered very deeply, and for that she has my sympathy, but little empathy. I have no conception of how it must feel to lose a child, and for some reason, I put the thought from me. Olivia continues to gaze at me, as though she can see inside me, and I fidget uncomfortably with the tubular frame of my chair.

Of course, all that Olivia is doing is passing on knowledge gained through pushing - three times - at the door that moves only one way. Two of her children might not have survived. She herself just cheated death with each of those births. She understands that some pain is qualitative, and that losing a child is utterly different in kind to other forms of suffering or bereavement.

I still don't know if she told me from some premonition, so that she could warn me, or whether she simply felt I needed educating. In any event, I understood, a year later, in the bone, in the marrow, what it was she tried to tell me that night. I know it now - completely, finally and forever.

Part Two

Early Pregnancy

9 Conception

If you follow the sunbeams
Through the valley of flowers
To the palace of the white queen
With its wide jade towers

I made this, I have forgotten
And remember.
The rigging weak and the canvas rotten
Between one June and another September.
Made this unknowing, half conscious, unknown, my own.

The women's group held a final social evening just after Christmas. We knew it would be the last I would attend, and I was showered with gifts and warmth and love. I remember Sylvia's parting comment about the group, "It's made all the difference, it really has," and despite my continued concern, when I looked at her, I thought she was probably right. Her diet continued, and she was still eating the equivalent of the vegetables out of the stew, but she had managed to become thinner while developing a softer, less angular look to her body. She was taking trouble with her appearance, and though that might be only superficial, it was a noticeable change. Sylvia had been to Nottingham and bought new, well-fitting leisure suits and had her hair cut in a page-boy style. She got changed now before meetings, whether her clothes were dirty or not. And although the depression sapped much of her strength, there was light behind her eyes that seemed firmly-established, and her words came firmer and faster. She wanted to look her best for us now, and for one person in particular - but that bit comes later.

I still have the stationery holder Olivia gave me as a parting gift, and its message, "for the new phase in your life," and as usual, she had summed it up exactly. I liked the image of a life as a moon, or a sea - constant, but living in all its phases. Sylvia's and Olivia's messages showed me that I was ready to move on. Of course, we could not know the enormity of the phase I was entering, or how deeply it would colour all others.

Actually entering the new phase was, however, somewhat protracted. Your dad started his new job in January in Eastbourne, but our first attempt to buy property had been abortive: we had nowhere to live. We put our furniture in storage and moved into a holiday bungalow while we tried again.

It was bleak, it was cold, it exuded condensation. It was even more lonely than Lincolnshire because, instead of looking out over endless fields, the view was of countless bungalows, just like ours, but empty. Your dad was at work all day, so I was suddenly thrown back on my fears of childcare. Constantly on the edge, I took your brothers out as often as possible and discovered new practical problems, like getting on a bus with two young children, a buggy and no help, or finding that virtually every shop doorway was three inches too narrow to accommodate a double buggy. And of course, I knew no-one. Inevitably, I fell back on my old mental trick of constructing a world in my head - a world with you, because that was my completion, living in a house we had done up ourselves. When your brothers were in bed in the evenings, I would find myself writing about this imaginary house, basing it very much on what I remembered of Tessa's or Jan's, describing every architectural and decorative feature. Sketches of houses also began to appear on the backs of envelopes. The ink on these pages constructed a dwelling as real to me as one made of bricks and mortar.

Gradually it became easier, as we joined mother-and-toddler groups and found the library. Also, Benjamin was old enough now to go to playgroup, and two mornings a week I would go into town, pretending I had only one child, as your dad asked incredulously when I told him this - "Pretend to whom?"

I could actually pretend, simultaneously, that I had one child, and that I also had my third child - my daughter, and "my" house. One fantasy related to short-term control, the other to personal fulfilment. And now, the pendulum hardly swung at all from the "world with you in it," and this was cemented by a visit to my friend Lesley.

Lesley lived in Brighton. I had met her when my family had moved house shortly before my twelfth birthday. She is about eighteen months younger than me. Living three doors away from each other, and attending the same school, throughout our teenage years we had been inseparable, and had sometimes pretended to be sisters. With the onset of adult life, we had stayed in pretty close touch, and it had often happened that great events in our lives coincided. She had her first daughter, Vicky, in the same month that your dad and I got married, and her second, Stacey, a month after Benjamin was born. And then she had had a third daughter, Lisa, about the time of Sam's first birthday. It was one of those friendships that always seemed to resume where it had left off, even if we did not meet for years.

One day, your dad had a meeting in Brighton, and deposited me and your brothers at her house for the day. Although her first exclamation when she saw me was "You've gone curly!" (I'd had a perm, in perhaps yet another attempt to be someone else) within a few minutes of us being together, we were the same people we always were with each other. Everything about Lesley's features is straight - her bobbed glossy brown hair, her nose, her teeth, her white neck, her legs. She gives the impression of making a complicated life easy. With the children, she seemed very laid back, and although they got into mischief, nothing ever seemed to get on top of her. I had lost Sylvia, Olivia, Tessa, Jan - back in an urban environment, I needed someone else to be. With you, Louise, I could achieve the same degree of what appeared to be happiness, if I were Lesley, and had *my* third baby - my daughter.

Lesley and her husband Ian were also trying to sell their house, to get a much more upmarket one, in Hove. Now that he, like many early eighties professionals, had set up his own financial consulting firm, they were making a lot of money. On one level, it did not escape my notice that the most your dad and I could hope to negotiate for was a flat, that he had only just managed to get a job. But on another level - that of the fantasies in my head - at least I could get on with having the same number of babies as she had, and one day, I was certain, I would have my house. I still didn't know how. Somehow, it seemed only a matter of waiting.

Then one moment, jerking out of time, sent the pendulum to the other end of its arc, and kept it there. It was Sylvia's birthday, 25th February, and I decided to ring her, from a call-box near the holiday homes. I had taken your brothers out for the afternoon, and we were coming back to get tea ready. Through the grimy window of the call-box I could see them in their buggy, cheerful coats warm against the gathering cold and late winter sea-dusk.

We spoke, she in a Lancashire accent now tinged with warmth, about how much we were missing each other. Everyone in the women's group was fine. She must have asked about Benjamin and Sam. I can't remember that part of the conversation, but I do recall a sentence of ice-crystal clarity:

"Well, at least you've got them through babyhood, and that's the main thing."

"Yes, that's true." I looked at them again. Stoically still, they looked as though they had been sculpted. Whilst my mind had wandered elsewhere, they, and I, had been achieving. They had learned to crawl, walk, and develop language, while part of me hardly noticed. Benjamin was out of nappies and Sam soon would be. I had constantly anticipated the next phase of their development but now everything was in place. They had hair and teeth and the bones of their skulls had moulded together. What remained was only a continuation. We had done it. The pendulum, after all, had swung in time, and now the project was complete. In a moment it was wrenched to the other end of its arc. I could not start again, not even for you. I decided, after all, that I didn't want another baby.

So how, Louise, did you happen? The simple answer is that I didn't put my cap in. The understanding of the action - or lack of action - is inordinately complex - a knot of conscious and unconscious motives, some of which I feel ashamed to admit to, but know I must.

I know the night it must have been. Your dad and I were a couple who had been married several years and had young children - the greatest desire we usually felt at bedtime was for sleep. I never put my cap in unless it was certain we were about to make love, even though it meant temporarily interrupting the proceedings. To have put it in every night as part of my bedtime routine - as the family planning people advised - would have meant succumbing to a law of increasingly diminishing returns. But that April night, knowing there was no barrier between egg and sperm, I did not get up to provide one. Our lovemaking was a rounded, uninterrupted whole. Sperm met egg and, at that point at least, they lived.

Perhaps, like Sylvia's baby, you were conceived out of carelessness, which, in our case, would have amounted to a mixture of laziness and lust. "I didn't want another baby - I couldn't be bothered not to have one." "I didn't want another baby - I wanted you," as if either of these, like getting drunk at a party, exonerates us from personal responsibility, for accepting blame for the consequences of our actions. Those selfish motives may well have been there, yet now, I think it may be no coincidence that I became pregnant just six weeks after making the final decision about my fertility. I felt, at long last, in charge of my destiny, even beyond the need for contraception. As I prepared to receive your dad inside me, I thought, "It's all right, I don't want another baby."

Yet far deeper than my new feeling of control was awakening a new spirituality, of which I was scarcely aware, but which was, through your little life, to form one of the tenets of my existence: let the Spirit decide.

And from a knot of selfishness, lust, arrogance and awakening spirituality, you were conceived. We both are sorry.

10 The Doctor

The youngest she sighed and
The clouds drew away
And a hundred small fingers
Scratched their heads in dismay.

Footfalls echo in the memory
Down the passage which we did not take
Towards the door we never opened
Into the rose-garden. My words echo
Thus, in your mind.
But to what purpose
Disturbing the dust on a bowl of rose-leaves
I do not know.

It is a clear, cold, Saturday morning, a week later. I take some clean washing into my bedroom, sit on the bed and start to sort it into neat piles of ownership. But I cannot concentrate even on this mundane task. My eye is held by the sky - bleached fleeces driven eastwards over ice-blue taffeta, colours becoming more brittle as they dry in the razor wind. For some reason, I think of Olivia, and walk over to the window for a view of the sea. Beyond other bungalows it moves restlessly, ruched grey with white frills. Unconsciously, I put out my hand, in a soothing gesture.

Quite suddenly, I feel very tired - a peculiar, anaemic and yet suffocating tiredness. I sit back down on the bed and mechanically continue my task. I know this is not the chronic tiredness I already suffer from, that it is not caused by my interaction with external circumstances, but that it is organic: it echoes in my bones. I have felt like this twice before. Instinctively, my hand moves towards my abdomen. I am pregnant.

I want this knowledge, yet I am not ready for it. I want to push it away, and consider the implications later, but there is something practical I must consider. I wander out to your dad, who is playing on the floor with your brothers.

"I've just had this weird feeling that I might be pregnant," I say, putting my hand on his shoulder, "so I think I'd better stop taking those tablets, just in case." I am taking tablets for my back. I have had sciatica intermittently since my first pregnancy, and my recent return to full-time motherhood has exacerbated it.

"Yes, okay" He doesn't seem to take much notice, his attention still caught by his two actual children.

What might have been and what has been
Point to one end, which is always present.

In the middle of the following week I go to see Dr Jackson, the G.P. we have temporarily signed up with. A square-jawed, square-shouldered man, he always seems to wear a charcoal-grey, three piece suit. I explain the situation in the matter-of-fact manner his appearance seems to elicit. In turn, he presents the facts as he understands them: that, even if I am pregnant, I have probably taken the tablets too early to make any difference. Then, apparently remembering earlier visits I have made with your brothers, he asks,

"Your children aren't very old, are they?"

"No," I admit, "the elder one is just three ..... the little one isn't two yet."

"Did you plan this pregnancy?"

Silence. Only the minutest silence, while I take in the enormity of the question now settling on his pink emulsioned walls, Lowry prints, and the photo of his children on the desk. The actual answer is easy to frame - I am still at the stage where I don't want another baby - but I still own the anguish and unfulfilled longing of the past year, like junk saved for a jumble sale. I know there is doubt in the eyes that smile at him as I reply,

"Not exactly."

Now it's his turn to frame a ponderous silence which he concludes with "What do you want to do about it?"

From the tone of our voices we could be speculating on the number of stones on Eastbourne Beach, but now, the silence is truly momentous. His three carefree children smile out at me from their paddling pool. We are considering the death sentence on a being I have wanted then executed, times without number, for over a year - a being who might not even have been conceived. When I eventually reply, part of me looks on. I do not know what I am going to say, yet when I speak, I feel as though I am repeating something rehearsed.

"I'd defend to the death any woman's right to abortion on demand," I reply. I am, after all, delivering Olivia's speech. "But," I went on, "I couldn't knowingly bring myself to destroy my own child." I had not even known I thought this.

"Then I don't think you should." He smiles in that knowing way of many doctors, inviting them to be your confidant. "Of course, it has to be your decision. No-one else should make it for you." He glances beyond me for a few seconds, through the vertical blinds, to shiny red-roofed houses opposite, then sighs.

"Quite a few years ago - not long after I qualified - I worked in an abortion clinic. Psychologically, the women split into two types. There were those you knew would be fine - they were totally convinced that was what they wanted. But there were also those you knew would carry a burden of guilt, for probably the rest of their lives. Despite knowing that what they had done was for the best, they would look on themselves as having destroyed their own child. Often, they had been pressured into the abortion."

I think of Sally, her control, her mental balance. I think of Lynne and all that wasted love. And I think, most poignantly, of Sylvia, who thought she could handle guilt better than post-natal depression, and how no-one should ever have to make that sort of choice. I picture her in her new clothes and new haircut, continuing to get thinner, and remember her once saying she would like not to be flesh at all, but a spirit of the air. And I wish, not for the first time, that I could hold the chrysalis of her unhappiness while she struggles free and flutters with fragile wings.

There is a profound sense in which Lynne's and Sylvia's babies are as real to them as Amber is to Olivia, and, because of the past year, you are as real as that to me. I know that, if I am pregnant, to end that deliberately would mean a grief I could not consciously seek. I think of your dad, and how I have no idea how he is going to react, but how I will have to be strong if he puts pressure on me. Somewhere in my womb I feel a flicker of protective tenderness towards you.

There is a complex and tortuous chasm between knowing you cannot destroy and actively wanting. I had not yet begun to want, but the first decision was made. In the event, you were taken from me, and I have other guilts to live with, but not that one. Probably I was already carrying a damaged child. But that, at least, is not my responsibility. I own only the consequences.

11 Discovery

From out of the sun a
Giant gull came flying
And the children got ready
To sit on its wing

On Friday, 22nd. April, 1983 - my birthday - your dad, your brothers and I left our temporary accommodation. The new season was approaching and we were no longer welcome at the holiday park. We had managed to buy a flat in St. Leonards-on-Sea, and that was the day we could pick up the keys. But our furniture was still in storage somewhere in Lincolnshire. Your dad had booked two weeks holiday to get it sorted. For the first of those weeks, your brothers and I were going to stay with his parents in Birmingham.

Having collected the keys from the estate agent, we had a look round the empty flat. It was another clear day, and we saw the flat at its best. It had been converted from a square-ish, semi-detached, pebble-dash Edwardian residential house. The two original rooms - the lounge and main bedroom - retained their spaciousness, with huge bay windows. The newly-created rooms were well-designed, and blended in effectively. And although classed as a ground-floor flat, the house was built on a slope so that the bedrooms were actually one floor up, the main one, with its bay window, commanding a view of the sea. The red kitchen was very poky, but well-arranged, and, as a friend later remarked,

"You've either got space to eat in a kitchen or you haven't. And if you haven't, it's pointless having one that's almost big enough." I thought of my struggles with doorways and a double buggy.

and now I might
As happy be as earth is beautiful,
Were I some other

It was a good flat. Had I been more at ease with myself, it would have been perfect. It was the home you should have come back to.

Before we set off for Birmingham, I bought some Lil-Iets. I actually thought now that a period might be going to come. I felt ratty, bloated and as if I were going to bleed. I didn't want to be stuck in Birmingham without tampons: care of bodily functions had never been the easiest conversation between me and your grandparents. Also, seeing the flat, especially on my birthday, had temporarily relaxed me and given me new hope: whilst I had an existence of my own I didn't need a baby. Pregnancy was not a physical condition. It was a state of mind.

However, by the Wednesday of the following week, the Lil-lets remained in the drawer, still sheathed in their polythene wrapper. I no longer felt bloated. I did feel ratty but I knew that was from months of broken sleep rather than a pre-menstrual hormonal imbalance. I certainly no longer felt as if I were going to bleed. Pregnancy seemed the only explanation. But when I thought back to my previous pregnancies, I didn't really feel like that either.

Caught in the form of limitation
Between un-being and being.

And that was how I experienced most of the pregnancy - not as a fullness, but rather as an absence, a void. Despite all evidence, particularly in the later stages, that I was going to have a baby, I often felt as though I wasn't. The initial absence was only of blood, but it led inexorably, despite your moving in my swollen abdomen, to an absence of life itself.

This may be part of the reason that I felt nothing when I actually bought a pregnancy test. I think too that, having now surrendered control I was experiencing the apathy of resignation. Just let it happen - whatever it may be. I am worn out with trying to decide for myself. All the same, I desperately needed to know if the world would be empty of you, or have you in it. Just five days after buying the Lil-Iets, I found myself in another chemist's, with your brothers and your granny, furtively looking at pregnancy tests while her attention was taken elsewhere. I hid my chosen test under a pack of nappies in order to pay for both, just as she returned. If she was gobsmacked by the price of nappies as displayed on the cash register, she didn't say anything. We left the shop together, struggling, as usual, with the buggy and the door.

Pregnancy tests have come a long way since then: my surreptitious investigation of the pack when we got home revealed that this one involved weeing into a tube wide enough to accommodate an anorexic caterpillar, and doing amazing things with mirrors. The instructions also told me to do an early morning sample, since that would be more accurate. However, you could do two tests - and I didn't want to wait. So, placing books strategically on top of a chest of drawers, I carried out the test and waited. Nothing. My urine resolutely refused to change.

But I knew that the test didn't tell me I wasn't pregnant - only that it hadn't registered. Rather than accepting the test, I was convinced that it was wrong- and that my fate was held in the balance until it came right - no matter how many tests it took.

I did not need to go to such inordinate lengths, though. This was a time when Sam was waking me at five each morning, or earlier. The following morning I set up the second test before taking him downstairs and returned to it after a tense half hour. Without disturbing the fluid I moved it towards the steely dawn light, then peered up towards the bottom of the test tube, where an almost imperceptible ring was beginning to darken.

Yes! I punched the air, miming my rush of excitement and sense of achievement so long awaited. All the negativity dissolved as the daylight came. At last. At last, my daughter was going to come to me. I feel elated yet also at peace: something momentous and irrevocable has been decided. It happens through me: I am the instrument. You have been called into being and that has ended all that I can do.

Later, I also had more reason to feel glad that I confirmed the pregnancy as early as I could: because of my secret knowledge, Louise, we were together in spirit as well as body for the longest time that we could be. Time spent unaware of your little lightless life would have been precious time truly wasted.

12 Worcester

They waved to the raindrops
As they circled o'er the trees
The wind tossed their hair high
Flashing gold on the sea

Part of the way in which I loved your dad was to need his approbation in a way in which
he did not need mine. That need was a weak warp thread woven into the fabric of what
appeared to be an equal marriage. One of the things I would most have wanted for you was the
capacity to love without fear.

It is the following Friday night. I wait eagerly by the door for him to arrive: not just
because we have spent a week apart, but mainly because I am desperate for some hint of
approval now that he knows about you. It has not been an auspicious beginning. The previous
evening, over the phone. I told a convoluted story of trying the two tests.

"The first one was negative," I said, to which he replied "yes," in a way that suggested
there couldn't be any doubt and he didn't really know why I was doing a test anyway. "But the
second one wasn't." I had burbled on, trying to keep the excitement from my voice. If there was
any reaction, it was a dull "oh," like a heavy book dropped on carpet, defying further discussion.

Even on the night after Amber's birth, I don't think I had made it really clear how much I
longed - at times - for this baby, and for how long I had wanted it, because if he said no - as he
did - he would be aware of the extent of his control. Our dreams make us vulnerable to those
who can decide if we achieve them: our disappointments, to anyone who has knowledge of
them- who knows that we can hurt. So far, he has been, to some extent unknowingly, the arbiter
of the dream and of its disappointment. Now he is neither. He has lost control, but I don't feel it
has been passed to me: it is out there somewhere, in a muddy no-man's land, unclaimable. And I
am afraid. Intellectually I know that I am carrying half his genes and that he too bears
responsibility. But at no stage do I actually feel this. I can share neither the wanting nor the
unwanting with him. If I admit there are times when I don't want the baby, he may put pressure
on me to abort the pregnancy. Yet any admission of desiring this baby is a reminder of his loss of
control. I am committing the sin of wanting the baby - or at least, of not going through the
unwanting process with him. I am a lost child, for whom there is no forgiveness. I am very
lonely, carrying his only daughter. And I am losing one of my best friends.

But as I put the phone down heavily and felt again that flicker of tenderness in my
womb, I knew that, if it came to a choice, I would have to choose you and not him. I can feel that
strength inside me, coiled if needed, but I do not feel strong now.

I had hoped without hope that the knowledge that you were going to arrive would be all
that was needed: as soon as I look into his pale, unwelcoming eyes, I know that is not the case.
There is an invisible steel wall around him, forbidding the coming baby to be mentioned.

The following day, we made our way to Worcester on the train. His mum and dad had
offered to have your brothers for one night to give us a break. I can't remember why we chose
Worcester, or why we went on the train - perhaps the two are linked. I remember being
attracted by its associations with Elgar, and the idea, by extension, of being somewhere
quintessentially English. In some obscure way, I thought this would give me a sense of
belonging.

That visit is now a patchwork of memory. Most of the squares are lost to me now, but some remain vivid - the jolty little train, the slightly musty pink-walled bedroom, the lumpy bed, the rose-coloured candlewick bedspread, the cool damp weather. Four more of the squares are the things we did. They are the sorts of things we usually did when we visited any place together. We looked round the cathedral, watched some cricket, went to a Greek restaurant for a meal, went to see "Tootsie." Yet only the last was truly a shared experience. Often, your dad and I disagreed over films, but we both enjoyed this one. At the end of the evening, it gave me some uneasy hope.

Earlier, as I had walked round the cathedral, I had become aware that your dad was no longer with me - that I was on my own. Yet I also became aware that, though it was he who had wandered off, it was actually what I needed - that this could be a solitude of strength, not of fear. I looked up to the high vaulting, to the overarching windows, and felt profoundly blessed with the gift of life. I was alone with some concept of god and the child growing inside me. In the silence I had faced the altar, my hand on my womb, and prayed silently. The mother, the daughter and the spirit. My soul knew, as it had always known, that this was right. I had nothing to be forgiven for.

We came out of the cathedral and crossed over to the cricket ground. If your dad had had any kind of translational experience, he wasn't letting on. I had a strength that filled my veins, yet I didn't want recourse to it: I didn't want to have to choose. I just wanted him to accept, so that we could get on with our lives. Presumably I thought this best done by not attempting to breach that steel wall that was around him; by not alluding to the baby, by not upsetting him any further. So when we sat watching the cricket, cold creeping like a fog around our feet and legs, we sat apart, as strangers, staring straight ahead. The only comfort for our bloodless hands was our own pockets.

He semi-cleared the air over the Greek meal. I think I must have seized the moment to say something about you. For a few seconds that wall came down. He looked past my shoulder as I tried to meet his eyes, and said,

"I suppose I'll feel all right about it when it's here." Then the wall went round him again, and the moment was gone. I suddenly saw that in the long months of pregnancy ahead, there was an extra dimension to the waiting - waiting for you, and waiting for your dad to change his mind, if he ever would, waiting for him to hold you in his arms, accepting both you and his proud part in your being. But at least with the pregnancy, I knew how long the wait was likely to be.

There is one more square left to me. On the way home, I realised that I had lost a ring, given me by my mother. She had bought it from a friend and passed it on to me, partly because she knew I coveted it and also because it suited my short stubby fingers better than her long elegant ones. I liked it because the five diamonds were set into the band of gold, where they could sit, quietly perfect, unostentatious but rightly admired when looked at closely. I knew that, if I had not left it in the guest house, there was little chance of finding it. It was not its value - monetary or sentimental- that I would miss most. My ring was part of me. For many years it had been one of the breakwaters that shored up my identity, and now there was a gap where seawater could flood in and the shingle bed be utterly changed.

I know that my foundations are becoming stronger, but I don't know how long that will sustain me if I have to begin rebuilding the edifice.

13 St. Leonards

They came to the castle
And there they did fall
And they saw all the sadness
Through the crystal wall

Your children are not your children.
They are the sons and daughters of Life's longing for itself.
They come through you but not from you,
And though they are with you yet they belong not to you.

You may give them your love but not your thoughts,
For they have their own thoughts.
You may house their bodies but not their souls,
For their souls dwell in the house of to-morrow,
which you cannot visit, not even in your dreams.

The following Friday, exactly two weeks after my thirty-second birthday, we celebrated Sam's second. There had been some doubt as to how much he would enjoy it. When we got back from Worcester he wasn't well, and had a rash on his chest and tummy. We went to your grandparents' G.P. and he said that it could be German Measles. He couldn't be sure, as many allergies exhibit the same symptoms. I knew I was immune to German Measles, but at the same time I felt uneasy about the contact - a superstition, with no reason behind it. Knowing this, I pushed it to the back of my mind and concentrated on nursing Sam. Like most young children, he slept off the illness after a couple of days and was well able to enjoy his cake and candles.

At two, he had the soft, peachy skin of childhood, the small nose, the narrow red lips, but they carried an idea that they would hardly coarsen with the growing body, and this turned out to be the case. The same was true of his eyebrows, dark and delicate, and the translucent quality of his green eyes, framed with smooth dark lashes, a band of saffron yellow around his pupils. The white-blonde curls and chubby, dimpled limbs, of course, were sacred to that moment in his life, as was the gap between his two front teeth. For some reason, they had failed to grow properly. The gap made an otherwise typically child's face idiosyncratic and gave it cheekiness and character, preventing it being, for me, too achingly perfect.

He was also recognisably entering what is known, even to most lay people, as the "terrible two" stage. This was not exhibited as tantrums - all of my children were surprisingly placid - but with an ever-developing stubbornness, which dovetailed with a more obvious vulnerability. When we walked down the street Sam would say, "Mummy, people," and try and hide in my clothing. And though both these aspects of his behaviour may have been induced by entering that particular stage of childhood, I recognised that, like his delicate features, he would take them, translated by his development, into adult life. I saw in him the little Taurean that I had been, and still was.

You may strive to be like them, but seek not to make them like you. For life goes not
backward nor tarries with yesterday.

For so long, I had thought that there was nothing of me in my children. Now that I was discovering that there was, I was already pregnant with you - the child I had hoped would really be a little me. There was a sense in which I was quietly pleased about these developments in Sam's personality, but never did I feel that they had come too late, that had I had that knowledge earlier, I needn't have bothered with the pregnancy. No matter how like me my sons became, being male, they could never be my recreated self.

How much of myself was in my gender? I genuinely didn't know, but I did know, ironically, that I wanted a relationship with my daughter that transcended gender, that her femaleness would be the point through which I would reach her soul. And that from that point, we would each be free to go, to be our own people.

Of course, it is through your death, not your living, that I have set you free, and it is through your death that I have gained self-honesty. For, had you been like me in gender, I would not have let you go: I was too tiny inside. Like my mother before me, I would have tried to cling on, to stifle you. Please forgive me. The tears that run down my cheeks are very hot. Louise, I was not worthy. Only your death has made me so. Forgive my arrogance, my meanness of soul, my lack of self-knowledge.

There is a final irony: because your brothers are boys, I have no difficulty loving them completely yet being able to let them go, letting them be their own people, learning from them. I love the ways they are like me and the ways they aren't. And, in all probability, I could have "done right" by my children in this morally profound way had you not come into my life. Yet again, in my arrogance, I had never expected to have a malformed child who could not live. And that colours all perception of the meanings of my living children's lives. Simply because they live, I give thanks.

But Sam is almost two, and here I am, embroidered cloths of dreams beneath my feet, taking what control I can to make sure you have the right beginning. Having at last moved to St. Leonards, on the Tuesday after the Worcester weekend, I get a contact number for the local branch of the National Childbirth Trust, wanting to sign up with a doctor who would be prepared to give me a home delivery. Jayne Walton, a newly-qualified ante-natal teacher, gives me the name and address of a doctor based near the sea front in Hastings, and promises to send me a copy of the current NCT Newsletter.

In fact, our first visit to Dr Walker involved all of us, including your dad, at the end of his "holiday", sorting out the flat. For a few days - since moving, in fact - we had been suffering from small, red, itchy spots. The diagnosis was scabies, the remedy for which was to paint ourselves attractively from head to foot - particularly the genital area - with a whiteish liquid. At first, the doctor hadn't wanted to prescribe the solution for me, but when he looked it up in his records he found that it had "no contra-indications for pregnancy." Your dad painted the stuff on me that evening, after Sam's birthday tea. On one level I laughed with him, as we became increasingly like characters in "The Addams Family." On another, I felt a repeat of that uneasy feeling, as if I were doing something I shouldn't be.

"Don't be silly." I tried to take myself in hand, looking from my bedroom window the following day onto a hazy sea. "Be logical. The doctor in Eastbourne says the back tablets won't have harmed the baby. The doctor in Birmingham says Sam's German Measles won't have harmed the baby. The doctor here says the white stuff won't have harmed the baby. This really is a very lucky baby."

My hand went automatically to my womb, yet there was something I was not as ease with, something I could not put my finger on. Less and less was it not wanting the baby. When we had been to the new doctor, and I had told him of the pregnancy, his spontaneous reaction was "good," and that had answered the new strength in my soul, and I knew that it was. There were still waves of un-wanting, but they were steadily losing their force.

The following Monday was ante-natal day at the surgery, and I went for my first check-up. My blood pressure and urine were checked by Sister Lennox, who would monitor the pregnancy and deliver the baby at home, so long as the flat was suitable. Health-wise, I was perfectly normal, I was also examined by Dr Walker who, like Dr Jackson, also dressed in a sombre three-piece suit. He had dark straight hair, rather thick and untameable, a chalky complexion which always made him look tired, and, although he spoke, as my mother would have said, "beautifully," his voice had a gravelly edge to it, as though he needed to clear his throat, or as if it too was in need of a rest. He also declared that everything was fine. Of course, at that stage, it was only me and not you that they could gain information about.

Because I was booked for a home delivery, I could not have the routine scan that I had had with your brothers. Basically, if you weren't going to have the baby in hospital, you weren't entitled to the use of their equipment at an earlier stage. In a way I felt disappointed that I would not "see" you at this earlier stage, but in another I felt it was right not to intrude on the mystery of a newly-created life. And there was no other sense in which not having a scan could be a problem. Everything was fine.

14 Toddler Group

A princess lay sleeping
So gentle and kind
Whilst her prince took to battle
With his confused mind

Urban living would, I recognised, at least give me the opportunity to feel less isolated, but it was in what I might at the time have considered an unlikely place that I met two women whose significance in my life - and to yours – is, and will always be, pivotal.

On Sam's birthday, after we had been to the doctor's and got the anti-scabies lotion, your dad took Benjamin and Sam for a walk and discovered the mobile library. It visited our road at the same time every week, and it was to become an important part of our routine once your dad was back at work. By chance - if there is such a thing - a woman popped in for a chat with the librarian - one of her friends. This woman, wife of the vicar of our local church, was setting up a mother (they never seemed to be parent) and toddler group, and was on the lookout for recruits. Seeing Benjamin and Sam, she gave your dad the details. The group met on Friday afternoons, two till four.

I remember the hall as a typical church hall - brown walls, unvarnished floorboards, dusty arched windows. A damp, unpleasant smell also emanated from the toilets, no matter how much they were bleached and cleaned. Yet it was one of the most relaxed and friendliest of groups, and that's partly why I hardly missed a session through the sorrows and joys of the three years we spent in St. Leonards. Even when your older brothers were at school, I had only one baby to concern myself with, and though the staple diet of toddler group conversations - "how long does he sleep for?" "does he eat much?" "how many teeth has he got?" - wore a bit thin, I stayed loyal to St. Andrew's toddler group. Set in Benjamin's, Sam's and my weekly pattern after our visit to the mobile library and looking at our new books together, it never quite lost its magic, remaining one of the highlights of my week.

But a far more important reason was Alison and Tina, who continued to be a substantial part of the magic even after Alison had moved away and Tina's toddler group visits had become very erratic. Unconsciously, as I realise now, I was looking for other women to be, now that Sylvia, Tessa, Olivia and Sally were no longer there, and, more importantly, now that I could no longer have a rural life that resembled theirs. My one contact with Lesley, significant though it was, was not enough to give me a coherent point of contact. That first Friday afternoon, I found the women who would.

I had thought that my feminism had stopped me thinking in stereotypes - at least, it was meant to have. Alison Archer was the woman that your brothers and your dad had met in the mobile library. He had told me that they had met the "vicar's wife," and when I met her I realised I'd been expecting a middle-aged woman in a "cardy", if not exactly twin set and pearls.

So it was with a mixture of shame and surprise that I met someone I immediately recognised as a chalky alter-ego. With the same complexion as Dr Walker, she was dressed, like Jan Moore, in the Clothkits dungarees and clogs that I aspired to but never seemed to get round to purchasing. Her hair was the same light-brown colour as mine, but thicker and straighter. And her eyes were blue and round, but where mine tended to grey, hers looked dipped in pallid watercolours - not unlike your dad's. She was slim too. For as long as I could remember I had hated not only my fatness but my silly red face. I had longed to look anaemic - had spent hours, years before, in fact, with white, and subsequently green, make-up, trying to achieve this effect. But I always looked like a rosy-cheeked person who was trying to cover it up, and eventually I abandoned the project. Like Helen Jones, Alison was attractive in an average sort of way. I should have remembered that, although I could imitate the trendy clothes and hairstyle, Alison Archer and I were not the same and that our destinies lay along different paths.

In one of our first conversations I told her about Sam's birthday, and then about the pregnancy. We were standing with a group of other women, and I realised after a while that I had unconsciously copied Alison's posture. I told them that I'd had the pregnancy confirmed that morning, which wasn't strictly true, but seemed an easier explanation. All the women, without exception, were thrilled for me, even though they hardly knew me, and this, coming on top of Dr Walkers declaration of "good," made me feel positively elated. It increased my strength - there was such power in women, and in their numbers. I knew I was chatting too much and too loudly, that I was "playing to the gallery," but I had never before felt so positive about you. Alison also said that she had recently suggested to Michael, her husband of seven months, that they try for a baby, and it seemed likely that we would go through the pregnancies reasonably concurrently.

Of course, I was asked the inevitable question about wanting a girl this time, after two boys. There was no way I could admit to these women that I'd only really become pregnant to have a daughter, to the strength of my disappointment should you be a boy - I could not lay myself open to people I hardly knew. I do remember - and have to own up to saying - that I didn't really mind, but a girl would be the icing on the cake. In other words, I made it sound as if your brothers were the main part, and you were only to do with appearance, with sugary sweetness - a finishing touch. Even as the words formed in my mouth, I could tell they did not feel right, but it was only later that I realised how indefensible they really were. People smiled reassuringly: in fact, I think I was reiterating an idea so culturally assimilated that it wasn't readily questioned. In my defence, I might have said the same had I already got two daughters and was trying for a son, but of course, that wasn't the case. For the second time that afternoon, I was forced to own up to attitudes I thought I had left behind.

After that conversation I went and sat down in the "magic circle" at the far end of the room. Some old carpet had been found, and rickety wooden chairs arranged in a circle near its perimeter. The circle contained old but sturdy toys for babies old enough to sit, crawl and take notice of them, but too young to join in the hurly-burly of car and tractor driving at the other end of the room, that your brothers were engaged in. Chatting mothers sat bolt upright in these chairs, arranged in clusters of various sizes around the circle.

One of these mothers, who had two people on her right but no-one to her left, was breastfeeding a very young baby. Still intrigued by young babies, and anticipating having one again myself now, I sat beside her in the empty chair. She was talking to the women next to her, saying that the baby was her third child, that it had been a mistake, but that she was not finding it as hard to cope as she had feared. When I started to join in the conversation, I also found out that her second child, Callan, would not be two until July. In addition, this woman, whom I had now discovered was called Tina, gave me some heartening information.

"Nick - my husband - certainly didn't want the baby. We set up the test in my study, on some books." Shades of how I had worked, and felt, but I noticed, with a pang, the use of the word 'we'. "And then this ring formed, and Nick kept saying, 'It couldn't possibly be wrong, could it?' Of course I knew it couldn't. I couldn't get rid of the baby, so I gave him time to get used to the idea. In the end, he did."

I wanted to ask how long it had taken, but for once, took a more pragmatic approach. After all, this Nick and your dad were not the same person, and presumably Nick could feel that he and Tina were in an unwanted situation together, in a way that your dad couldn't with me. Also, I realised that if Tina told me how long it had taken Nick to accept the baby, I would probably wait for that length of time for your dad to accept you, which would be completely invidious. What did give me heart, though, was knowing that, now baby Dominic had arrived, and was a few weeks old, his dad loved him like his other children.

There were other things that attracted me to Tina, that made me want to accept her invitation to call round "anytime." It wasn't just my ever-threatening sense of isolation, which made me want to be with someone - anyone - at any time of the day or night. In all her gestures and expressions, especially the proverbially enigmatic smile that never seemed far from the edges of her lips, I was recognising, in some important part of me, that I was encountering a soul mate, albeit one a good deal less timid than me ... one without a neurotic need of external structure. At one stage, Tina looked across at her oldest child, now four, who was playing with Benjamin and Sam at the rowdy end of the hall.

"I trained as a teacher too," she told me, in response to me giving some background information about myself. "But I became pregnant with Osheen during my PGCE year, and got married. Although I was able to finish the course, I couldn't do the following year- my probationary year. I quite enjoyed the training. I was in the school in Croydon that DH Lawrence taught, and the men there were dead hip and thought they were really radical and they were getting English education sorted out. It was quite good fun. One day I might go back and do my probationary year."

She smiled enticingly, her slightly protruding teeth showing to good effect, framed by a wide, red mouth. She talked very naturally to everybody, and although her clothes were somewhat avant-garde she seemed to blend in a lot more easily than I did, even allowing for the fact that I was new in the town.

"What did you do your degree in?" I asked, somehow knowing the reply before it came. After all, she had known about DH Lawrence, and although I no longer subscribed to his views - reading Kate Millett had put an end to that - I still felt touched by the passion of that formative reading.

"English literature."

I had, after a long, long time, chosen to read History rather than English at university, feeling that I needed a core of factual information, however it might be filtered, to interpret and analyse. But it had been a tough decision and I had gone to a university - Sussex - that had enabled me to incorporate that love of my life into my studies.

I looked at Tina's long mahogany-coloured hair, backcombed at the crown in a way I hadn't seen since the early sixties. She had high cheekbones like Sandie Shaw, although her face had a chubby quality to it and rosy cheeks like mine. Her eyes were a pure cornflower blue, framed by long dark lashes, but she tended to screw them up slightly when she talked to people, as if light was rather too much. Much of her body, like Alison's, was slender, with narrow hips, but retained the luscious rounded breasts and stomach of childbearing. The angular patterns on her translucent dress again suggested perhaps a fifties culture, but this was somehow because Tina was not going to be circumscribed by fashionable ideas, rather than because she was fixed in the past. Tina had the inner confidence to pick and choose from a variety of sources to create a synthesised image.

The name Osheen, she told me, had come from an Irish legend retold by Yeats. Tina was really living her life, freely, breaking the unspoken rules where necessary in order to do so. If

Alison was my physical alter ego, Tina was my spiritual one. It was because I sought to bring them to me, by making myself like them, that I caused myself, later, unnecessary pain, pain they would never have chosen to inflict on me. It was only as I could let them go - in the same way that I had to let you go - and rebuild myself, that I could not only forgive, but truly accept and love our differences as well as our similarities.

15 Emily and Claire

The clash of bright metal
Brought the children fear
But their cloaks of blue satin
Dried up all of his tears

And the children in the apple-tree
Not known, because not looked for
But heard, half-heard, in the stillness
Between two waves of the sea.

Sister Lennox came round to the flat the day after my first ante-natal visit to the doctor's, to check that it was a suitable place for birth. It did well. The bedroom was large, and near the kitchen and bathroom. The only difficulty she envisaged was the low bed, which your dad had purchased from Habitat shortly before I met him, and which we still considered quite hip. She gave me quite a formidable list of things needed for the delivery. Most of these are lost to memory now, but I do remember, that, for some reason, masses of brown paper was required. I decided to build the supplies up gradually - there was plenty of time.

There would also be plenty of time, I thought, to build on my relationship with Sister Lennox, which had got off to a good start. In many ways, in her blue uniform, and with a slightly rounded figure, she was the archetypal district midwife - highly competent, highly experienced and at the same time compassionate. I noticed that quality in her amber eyes more than any other. Also, of course, in delivering babies at home, to women she had got to know well, and working for a doctor who condoned giving women choice in childbirth, she was doing not only a job she loved, but in a way that she had herself chosen, and that she believed in. I felt at the same time safe and excited about the delivery. For once, I was going to have a baby in the way I considered right, and I had superb medical support.

After our little tour of the flat, she asked how I had heard of Dr Walker. I explained about finding Jayne Walton's number in the NCT newsletter, and getting the information from there.

"Ah. Yes. I know Jayne quite well. She recently finished training as an ante-natal teacher, you know."

"Yes. She'd written about it in the newsletter. She said that the training was fascinating."

"I'm sure she'll be very good. Did you actually talk to her on the phone?"

"Yes," I replied slowly, to what seemed a rather strange question. "How did she sound? Only she hasn't been very well recently."

"She sounded okay" I was trying to remember any indication that the woman I'd spoken to had sounded less than well, but couldn't recall any. I wondered if Sister Lennox thought I was at best unobservant, at worse, downright uncaring. "No," I concluded, "she sounded fine."

"Good." Sister Lennox sounded far from convinced, but was obviously too professionally discreet to tell me what the trouble was. "Anyway, she should certainly be ready to resume ante-natal classes by the time you want them - if you think you will."

"Definitely." I had never before been in a geographical location able to benefit from NCT classes, and although I'd already had two babies, I wasn't going to miss out this time. And with the promise of meeting again at the clinic in a month, and mutual wishes of goodwill, she took her leave.

I was thinking about Jayne and her mysterious illness when the phone rang, and it was actually her. She sounded bright, cheerful, organised - those things I had heard before. If anything, perhaps there was a slight thickness to her voice, as though she had been crying some time before. But certainly, without Sister Lennox to alert me, it would have been imperceptible. She said that I may have noticed there was a coffee morning the following day in Hastings Old Town (I had) and that if I liked, she would give me and your brothers a lift. Stammering gratitude, I accepted.

I could easily equate the woman I had spoken to on the phone with the one who arrived on my doorstep next morning. She had a beaming smile and dimples in both cheeks, suggestive of easy friendship. Yet her eyes, though they, too, smiled, were stabbingly blue. Her direct look demanded honesty from me without compromise, and told me that I was meeting a woman who did not expect to be bullshitted or messed around with. It also told me that she would meet me with that same brutal honesty, and that the integrity of every moment mattered - that there was no time for playing games.

Her short hair was highlighted and swept back - it looked as if it had money spent on it regularly. Her white shirt and full summer skirt were plain cotton fabric but well-cut. At her side stood a four-year-old boy who was introduced as Barnaby. He had thick, shiny-white curls and his confident smile was a smaller version of his mother's.

Seeing Barnaby, who towered over Benjamin, it did cross my mind to wonder whether Jayne had thought of having more children, as she had clearly put a lot of personal investment into the NCT. It was pretty unusual for women without young children to maintain a high level of involvement in the organisation.

It was a beautifully delicate early summer day, with a childlike breeze that played with the world and its light. Leaves in gardens were translucently tender both in their size and juvenescent shades of green. We glided towards the sea front. Pools of white light glittered on the lulling pale blue surface of the sea. I was gently aware of the new life growing within me.

It is always crowded in the Old Town, and parking is a nightmare, so we stopped the car near the sea front and walked to the coffee morning. For me, it was a difficult walk, shrouded in confusion. If I had been then the person I am now, it would not have been.

We had been driving along the sea front when Jayne asked,

"Did Jean Lennox say anything to you about - my recent history?" "Well," I replied, anticipating some juicy information, "she said you hadn't been very well recently. I didn't like to pry."

Jayne's smile was slightly bitter and at the same time indulgent. "Typical Jean. That's very discreet of her. But it must have left you wondering."

"Well - yes."

I just about noticed Jayne draw breath before continuing.

"Jean Lennox was my midwife. Six weeks ago, I had twin daughters. They were born twelve weeks too early. Emily was the bigger of the two, and she was born first, but she lived for only a few hours. Claire hung on for about a week and then she died. They were lovely girls, and they were very pretty."

"Oh Jayne, I'm so sorry." Somewhere in my mind this sounded like the right thing to say, and I would say it now, but the inner meaning would be changed utterly. Now, it would mean, *even though I hardly know you, I will at least hold your hand, and perhaps put my arm round you, so that you know you are not alone, and I will support you through this in any way that I possibly can. I know that you are at the edge of human experience and I will join you there, not with my own burden, but to help you make sense of yours.* Then, those mumbled words were merely a cover-up for my own inadequacy and embarrassment. I wanted to say something appropriate, but simply didn't know what. I felt that I didn't have the reference points in my own life to say anything useful – ironically, now that perhaps I do, I realise that I didn't need them: that whatever I might have offered Jayne, as long as it was me, and it was genuine, would have been enough. But Jayne was still a virtual stranger and those are the most difficult of relationships for the bereaved. Our friends, and those closest to us, go through the tragedy with us - there is mutual mourning, and no holding back the tears and cuddles. Normally, though, we want choice about who we open ourselves up to, and grief denies us that choice. We must reveal our unhealable, gaping wounds, still at their most raw, to everyone.

But if that's hard, it's also far from easy, without a trained compassion, to have to see those wounds. We feel guilty for witnessing an obscenity, this total emotional violation of a stranger's life. We do not want to be implicated. I could understand how people cross to the other side of the road to avoid the bereaved. I may have been ashamed of myself, but that did not alter the fact that, as I walked in silence next to Jayne, that's what I wanted to do.

Suddenly, I could understand how people trotted out trite phrases of sympathy. If not quite the verbal equivalent of crossing over to the other side of the road, it was pretty close. Partly it is in the genuinely well-meaning, but mistaken notion that such phrases will provide comfort for the bereaved. More importantly, they provide comfort for the so-called comforter, steering the conversation back towards the optimistically trivial, and deflecting from the enormity of an experience that most of us cannot cope with, even vicariously. Any of the phrases that came to mind then, once uttered, might absolve me from any kind of emotional responsibility for this bereaved woman, and return us to a less problematic area of conversation. "You can always try again." "It was probably for the best." "I know how you must feel"

As I said, I'm not exactly proud of how I handled these moments, but at least I rejected each phrase in turn. I realised that Jayne wanted those children back, and that no amount of new ones would make up for her loss. I could see no way in which losing her daughters could be for the best, so it was highly unlikely that she could. Finally, as I had had to acknowledge with Helen Jones, I really had no idea what Jayne was going through, and it would be invidious to imply that I did. I mooched along, busying myself with my own children, being unusually paranoid about the busy road, and avoiding those achingly honest eyes. I knew now why she didn't waste time with games. I knew she deserved better, but did not know how to provide it. Eventually, we reached the High Street and could discuss the shop window displays - the time lapse doing the same job as perhaps the trite phrases would have done, but at least I hadn't fobbed her off.

It has occurred to me since, when I think of the things that are said to bereaved people and the way they are treated, it is as children. Again, it is kindly motivated. We want to lead people away from pain, so we metaphorically pat them on the head and say, "There there, you'll get over it," as if they have fallen over and scraped their knee. We become impatient if they do not appear to be "getting over it" within a limited time. Occasionally, we may even tell the bereaved that it is not the end of the world. But that's precisely what it is. The world, as the bereaved person knew it, has been shattered.

Though well-intentioned, this patronising attitude, this treatment of the bereaved as if they were little children, carries a savage irony since, in many ways, that is precisely what they are. Like children, they live totally in the present, for the past has changed irredeemably and the future - even tomorrow - is inconceivable. The bereaved have to begin to rebuild their lives again, but every brick that is put in place is knocked down many, many times before a single wall is built. Yet if they are patronised, and their suffering played down, the bricks will lay forever on the ground, spread randomly. They never will acquire the skill to build and see new patterns. Bereaved people are not taking a temporary break from the real world, with an aim to resuming normal service as soon as possible. Nothing is more real than human suffering. Regarded as temporarily broken human beings, the bereaved are somehow less than whole. In truth, they're actually going through a process of becoming more truly human, and therefore should command our respect and total support, not our patronising.

16 A Cot

The children held hands and
They spelled out her name
All the golden children
Became a golden chain

If you would indeed behold the spirit of death, open your heart wide unto the body of life.
For life and death are one, even as the river and the sea are one.

Apart from stark moments that I must include in this chapter I felt a lot more at peace about the pregnancy towards the end of those early weeks. Since I had seen Dr Walker, and perhaps more importantly, Sister Lennox, the pendulum had virtually stopped swinging. I had completely forgotten how special the medical attention could make me feel, and I welcomed it back like an old friend. That, as well as meeting women I related to, who were pleased about the pregnancy, melted my unwanting moments. And although I could not take Jayne's grief into my soul, I knew, in a detached way, that I was privileged to have a living child inside me.

My mood concerning you was like the sea that, with your brothers, I visited most days now: a succession of sunny days brought gentle movements. There were wavelets of not-wanting, but they were gentle, background waves only, being inexorably taken out by the tide's invisible force. When your dad was at home, I could still feel your being as a tangible knot dividing us, but when he was out of the house, I felt that knot dissolve.

So, with a new freedom of mind I focused more on the world-with-you-in-it scenario, and it felt more right than ever before. But while I acknowledged, even consciously, that there was little point now in creating fantasies empty of you, and that relieved a lot of inner tension, I also began to see clearly for the first time the almost superstitious power I had previously attributed to my own fantasies. I had wasted a lot of neurotic energy in feeling I had to decide, once and for all time, what my future would be, because I believed it would actually happen if I visualised it decisively enough.

I'm not denying that visualisation can be a useful psychological tool. Tina's husband studied it intensively and produced some good literature on the subject. But I do think you have to be created first - to have a clear inner idea of where you're going you need to know where, and who, you are, and I didn't. Visualisation may be able to help you achieve what you want, but first you have to know what that is, consistently. Above all, visualisation needs to embody the principle of gentle change: I wanted fantasies immutable as marble. I tried to use it to find out what I wanted, while all the time my life was lost to me. Knowing that you were inside me, I was gradually starting to reclaim that life.

That's what made it hard when, without warning, I suddenly realised I wanted you dead. I did not want the pregnancy, the baby, more endless washing - anything. Since seeing Sister Lennox and acquiring the formidable list of things needed for the home delivery, my mind had happily filled itself with plans for your arrival in the world and subsequent upbringing. Now, nothing worked. There was still time for an abortion. I knew that Dr Walker was out of the question, but Dr Jackson in Eastbourne might be prepared, if only I could sound convincing enough. I believed I could. The tidal wave of hatred and intense loathing would, I felt, make any feelings of remorse I might be tempted to feel totally irrelevant. I did not want you, and I believed nothing could ever make me want you again.

I loathed myself too, for the plans I had been making for both of us. In my new, easier feelings about myself and you, they had seemed part of a statement about what I wanted to achieve now with regard to having children - a culmination of putting those principles into action. Now they seemed at the best irrelevant to my life, and at the worst, mushy. Apart from the fact that they were always about a girl, I realised, in a stabbing moment of self-honesty, that they could be about any girl, so long as she came to me. But I felt my hatred, my longing to be rid, was directed only at you. It could never be deflected anywhere else.

The actual abortion I contemplated with frightening precision but there was one thing that stopped me making the phone call. It was the knowledge that I would have to lie to all the people who already knew about you. Yes, I believed now that I could destroy my own child - but I did not want anyone else knowing about this heart of my darkness. I imagined telling each of them in turn, with stunning clarity, that I'd lost the baby. It was as if I were looking through the wrong end of a telescope.

It was your dad who, in his own continued hostility, reminded me we were on a spiral, and that this tidal wave was part of an established pattern, like putting too much ink on a silk screen print. Despite my somewhat unstable inner life, I had not thought it unreasonable when I got ratty one morning because one of the kids had spilt some milk in the bedroom. (The fridge was in our bedroom because it wouldn't fit under the kitchen unit, and that was pissing me off as well.) I then got cross about some dropped toast, and I can remember his voice now as he said,

"If you carry on like this, you can forget all about having this baby."

I know I said nothing. I was aware of Benjamin looking at me, uncomprehending, while Sam carried on with his breakfast. For an instant I wondered if my husband had been able to read my thoughts and picked them up when I was at my most negative. Then the threat sank in for a second time. I stood very still while part of my mind looked on and wondered why I wasn't trembling, and another part told me that this is what it feels like to be petrified. The idea of abortion, which I had considered so seriously, was now a frivolity I had allowed myself while off guard against the real situation. Suddenly, it was me and the baby against whatever he could do to threaten either of our existences, but this time I was too scared even to feel protective towards you. You and I were the same flesh, but we were equals, facing him together. I walked out of the room, lifting my heavy, brittle feet slowly. My heart had started to beat again. And in yet another corner of my mind, I wondered if, after this, you would ever begin to move.

A few days later, as your brothers and I were just leaving home to go and see Jayne, we had to go back in the house again because Mummy felt a bit sick. Probably my mood of the previous week had been a forerunner of the sickness, or certainly due to hormonal changes, unrecognised because not all of me was ready to move on. I remember feeling relieved, while I was throwing up, that your dad was not there, in case that might be construed as "carrying on like this." As well as not mentioning you now, I went out of my way to minimise the normal effects of nausea, sickness and tiredness that early pregnancy usually had on me.

Fortunately, as I considered at the time, I did not have to make too much of an effort. Nausea I could make an effort to disguise, and I always felt tired anyway - no difference there. After our delayed journey to Jayne's house, I think I was only sick a couple of times in those early weeks, and that was easy to conceal. I had thrown up abundantly in the early stages of both my previous pregnancies, and this confirmed to me that, since this was so different, I must be having a girl this time. Of course, it never occurred to me that, for me to feel O. K. in early pregnancy was actually abnormal. It seems now that I have to pay a high price in terms of my own health to produce a healthy baby. It was only at the end of this pregnancy that there was to be a lot of pain - but it was of a totally different kind.

Friday evening. I am sixteen weeks pregnant. It is a normal Friday night, in the sense that we have done our weekly shopping at the out-of-town Tesco's and collected fish and chips for our supper on the way home. While we are eating it, your dad suddenly says,

"A woman at work was saying that her baby's just growing out of his cot, so I said we might be interested. There's bedding as well. She did say that the cot needs a lick of paint, but we could soon fix that."

"Great." With deliberation I add more ketchup to the side of my plate, although I have plenty already, and try and act as normally as possible while I absorb the impact of what he is saying. He is not only prepared to make practical arrangements, which means he accepts that we are going to have a baby, but to tell at least one person at work. And since he is not the kind of person to confide things to people he does not know intimately, I assume that, in his office, this is now common knowledge.

I feel as if I am standing on the edge of the shore. The water is clear, with tiny waves of lace that break over my feet. To start with they are icy, but gradually they become warmer and my toes relax. At the moment I don't dare go any further in: somewhere out there I will be out of my depth, and I'm not sure where the place is.

I put the ketchup bottle down.

"Of course, we are going to need a cot. Find out if she's got anything else going cheap." I smile tentatively, and when I look questioningly at him, he looks back. I can't remember the last time we had intimate eye contact, and I realise how much I've missed him, and what I risked giving up in order to have you.

Your brothers say they've finished and ask to leave the table. Again, in what feels like the first time in a long time, your dad and I indulge in one of our less attractive habits, which we call "vultching." Basically it means helping ourselves to any of the boys' leftover food. We share it out between us. I realise that I am still quite hungry, and I have quite a pool of tomato ketchup to dip into.

"After all," I suddenly allow myself to think, "I'm eating for two now."

I still daren't articulate this thought, but I am aware of eating with more freedom and enjoyment than I have for many weeks, and we finish off the chips together.

Friday night. It must be exactly fourteen weeks since your conception, since I am sixteen weeks pregnant. (That particular piece of mathematical gynaecology has always intrigued me.) One advantage of my being pregnant is that we do not have to think about contraception. I would not say that to date, the pregnancy has affected our sex life. Although you were the product of that, there was a conflict to be resolved that became separate from our physical need of each other. This night, though, as we make love, I feel the three of us are together. I no longer have to exclude you from my thoughts in order for you dad and I to share each other, and you, completely.

One week later, I feel a soft movement in my tummy, like butterfly's wings. It is the right time. I no longer consider myself just pregnant. Your dad and I are going to have a baby.

17 Childhoods

It lies on the white throne
In a magic place
With a tunic of velvet
And a gown of white lace

Meanwhile, and apart from the implications that your hidden being had on me, your dad and my relationship with him, I continued to look after your brothers and to keep the flat as tidy as I could, and reasonably clean. (Although cleanliness may be hygienically more desirable, it was how tidy the place was that people would notice first.) Within the confines of the flat, motherhood did not get any easier, and in a specifically emotional way that I want to look at in a bit, it got more difficult.

I continued to be virtually obsessed by the writing I wasn't doing, and yet I could not know that this had more to do with my perception of myself as a mother than with the situation itself. When I returned, some years later, to full-time teaching, I still felt a need to write but it was based on the knowledge that this was the only medium for fulfilling that part of my creativity. While your brothers were little, writing was not simply my only escape, and a chance to do something that occupied my mind as well as my time: it gave me a link, albeit a tenuous one, with the outside world. Most importantly, the patterns of letters on paper gave me a self. Yes, you write for an imagined audience, and therefore play a part, but at least I had the choice of writing things that I myself would choose to read. When I had signed up for the part of "mother," I had failed to realise how demanding it would be, what a long run it would have, or its potential to destroy my flimsy identity. Neither did I realise the changing nature of those demands, even as your brothers grew and developed, and it is only now, looking back from the vantage point of a decade, that I realise their impact now.

I don't think I realised it at the time because most of what was happening took place on a continuum: in the same way that we swapped night nappies for getting Sam up before your dad and I went to bed ourselves, and watching him wee while still totally asleep, or tying up shoelaces instead of pulling on bootees, the emotional changes like the "terrible two" syndrome were still rooted in the little personalities that I had known and nurtured since babyhood. I knew and recognised these children - they were simply the same little people at different ages, and as I have said, Sam had much of the same stubbornness and vulnerability as his mother.

Also, prospective parents know that, with children's development, while the physical side gets easier, the emotional side becomes more difficult, as the child has to learn to accept that they are not at the centre of the universe. I read copious amounts of advice on how to handle these conflicts. Yet nowhere did I see any reference to how my children's emotional rawness, vulnerability and anger would bring those qualities right to the surface in me. Effectively, we were three toddlers, although I was the one who arranged things. Neither was I prepared for the intense pity I felt when they were emotionally injured in some way, whether by me or someone else.

I can remember three episodes that show so clearly how we were all trying to make sense of our lives, and precisely how much we were investing in doing just that. The sequence of these events is lost to me, but I know they took place during those early months of the pregnancy. Part of the routine of our lives was to collect the child benefit on Mondays. With that money, I would of course buy some food, and sometimes, I treated your brothers to a drink in a cafe. One particular Monday morning I realised I had lost the child benefit book. In the state I existed, this represented far more than the loss of the book, or even making different arrangements for buying food: a great gash had been torn in the defences of my existence. I sat down heavily on the edge of the bed and cried: the baby, stilt, felt like a weight in me. I repeatedly searched my basket, an increasingly futile gesture, and then cried with that futility. Eventually Benjamin wandered in. My distress was matched only by his own, in seeing me so upset. I completely forgot to address him as a three-year-old.

"I've lost my book," I sobbed, "I've lost my book." I could hear my voice was unusually shrill. A few seconds later he was back, clutching a copy of "Mr. Greedy Goes Shopping," which he held out to me.

"Here's a book, Mummy, here's a book," he said desperately, tears coming to his large blue eyes. I have noticed since, in my own despair and attempts to make sense, my tendency to repeat phrases, just as I did when upset as a child, and just as my own children did.

My frustration gave way to pity. Like me, he wanted to do so much and could do so little, but he was so much smaller than I was. I could not begin to explain why I was still crying, and crying so much more steadily than before. It was not hard to lift him onto the bed next to me and explain that this was not the right kind of book, and we would have to go to the post office and see about getting another one. It was much harder for me to change our plans for the day: their immutability was one of the main sources from which I attempted to draw security.

The next incident took place one lunchtime. We were going to have yogurt for pudding. The new four-packs of yogurts had just come out. I fetched a new pack from the fridge, breaking them up into separate yogurts as I came through into the front room. Benjamin, always an equable child, chose one calmly, but Sam was not prepared to go along with this. He wanted to separate the pots himself, and could not accept that it could not be done. I tried to pretend that they had magically stuck themselves together, but of course, as soon as he took them from my hand they separated again, without that satisfying crunch that he wanted, and now, I hadn't just separated his yogurts, I'd tried to deceive him too.

All he wanted now was real magic that would put them together again - and I would have done anything to be able to provide it. I'd felt the frustration mounting in me, but there was little I could do to check it. Snatching up the remaining three yogurts, I made for the nearest wall that wasn't papered - I had the presence of mind to do that - and threw them at it as hard as I could. Then, slamming as many doors behind me as I could, I rushed out of the flat.

I only walked a short way down the road. I knew that if they hurt themselves then, it would be my fault, but I simply could not go back in to them. Although Benjamin had had nothing to do with it, I had no feelings for either of them. I contemplated just leaving, and hoping they would be all right until your dad got home. Then I stopped walking away, and without noticing what I was doing, I was returning in the direction of the flat, but I was gliding. Only my mind seemed to be working; my body did not know what it was doing. I don't know how long I sat on the wall outside. This is not what I meant at all. This is not it, at all. I could only go back in when I felt able to face the spilt yogurt - the least of the things I had spilt.

I still felt nothing as I opened the door again. The flat was quiet - it too felt pregnant. Then I heard sobbing, coming from their bedroom. Soundlessly I moved towards the door and listened outside. I heard Benjamin's voice, so desperately poignant now because he was trying to deal with his own distress as well as his younger brother's.

"It's alright Sam," he was saying between sobs. "You'll be all right. I'll look after you. You'll be all right. I'm here."

I opened the door, and they both looked at me. Benjamin had both his arms round Sam, who looked confused as well as upset. For a second, they looked frightened. All the feelings I had been holding at bay to protect myself now rushed in, destroying all barriers. We all cuddled together on the bed. I sobbed for a lot longer than they did, and it was a long time after that that I remembered to clear up the yogurt.

The third incident also had to do with my need to escape, and the sheer impossibility of it. In the evenings, I could escape into my writing. During the day, I would sometimes try to escape and find myself - whoever that was - simply by removing myself from your brothers for a while, once I knew they could be safely left. Once, when I had wandered into my bedroom, and Benjamin had followed me, I asked, in sheer frustration, why he had to keep following me about.

"Because I love you Mummy, and I want to be with you all the time." Having given me a straightforward fact from his world picture, he could understand neither my initial frustration, nor the hot tears that splashed onto his shiny, straight fair hair as I held him to me.

It's all over now, that time in our lives. We have all moved on. I have made other life choices: they are about to begin making their really important ones. They choose their own friends now and pursue their own interests. They do some things for me - perhaps they could do more - and I no longer have to do everything for them. I longed, perhaps more than most mothers, for us to get to this stage - for that to be over. But even I feel nostalgic, looking back, that we will never have that time again, that they will never again look so beautiful to me, that I will never again love them, as they loved me, with such desperate, vulnerable, intensity.

If I could, I would regret wishing it away and not enjoying it more. But that would only have been possible had I been someone else, and, although I had tried, I had found that was something I could not control. By the time I had become someone else, it was too late. And though I may have made a mess of your older brothers' early childhood, at least I do have it, and hold it, as a memory becoming more, rather than less, precious. It was not something offered, promised, and then snatched away.

My sword it lies broken
And tossed in a lake
In the dream I was told that
My princess would wake.

If I could not escape from my children, I could at least escape with them. While the background of those three storyboard pictures is the flat we shared, we actually spent as much time as we could away from it. It was well worth all the hassles involved in actually getting two young children ready to go out, although, of course, it was a good deal easier in summer anyway. We went for walks along the seafront, to the beach, or to the beautiful Alexandra Park- one of the most extravagantly landscaped urban parks there must be. I know that it was devastated in the 1987 hurricane, and I have not seen it since: it remains in my memory as an expanse of undulating mixed woodland that virtually bisected the town: I actually got lost in it once. On our visits out I could not really relax, since in all these excursions there were dangers, especially since both the boys - especially Benjamin - liked to wander off. But it felt mentally better to worry about them getting lost, falling in water or simply falling over. Real or imagined, these were at least threats from which I, as their mother, could protect them - I did not have to protect them from myself.

Also, just being outside lifted pressure from my chest. I could feel the salt air inflating my lungs, conveyed to me on the pale gold summer breezes.

Of course, these visits, vital though they were to my sanity and, by implication, the boys' overall well-being, could not provide what I craved more than anything else - the company of women. With the watercolour backgrounds of our trips out deepening to oils as we moved towards summer, these had to give precedence to the repeating stencil of things that other people, performing a crucial social service - at least for me - had provided.

The Friday jaunts up the road to St. Andrew's toddler group were supplemented by Monday afternoon trips to the Meet-a-Mum Association, or MAMA. That first NCT coffee morning, which I went to with Jayne in the Old Town, turned out to be the first of many. In the same way that Sylvia and I had always been to Women's Group meetings, I became something of a coffee morning groupie. Regardless of where in the town they were held, how far it was to walk or how many buses we had to catch, we were there.

Virtually any women would do in satisfying my need, but - and I admitted the elitist nature of this to myself only reluctantly - the most delicious stimulation was to be gained from contact with thinking women, and preferably those with similar interests to myself. The Women's Group had got me started, and although it had reached a natural end, I knew that, in some way, I had to go on from there.

All the organisations I've so far mentioned provided what I wanted to some degree: set up primarily for mothers with young children, they also contained some women who thought independently and wanted to change the way things were done. Yet while this was obviously true of the NCT and its laudable, and successful, campaigns to give women informed choices about their care in pregnancy, childbirth and beyond, this was the sole scope of its parameters. Intrinsically, of course, this was its strength, but it did mean that the organisation contained many confident, competent and, it must be said, middle-class women who were content with this single-issue campaigning and did not, or chose not to, consider that it might have any kind of challenging social and political ramifications. One of my best friends from about ten years before (Little Pete - whatever happened to him?) once said that you could find the same cross-section of intelligence on a shop floor as you could on a university campus. I found the same thing to be true of mothers' support groups, whether their base was from the immediate community - toddler groups - or served a population with more access to private transport - the NCT.

It was the previous year that had seen the rapid growth of CND membership, largely with the arrival of Cruise missiles, and although, in Lincolnshire, we had been well removed from the campaigning, it was an issue that I was becoming increasingly neurotic about. The December of 1982 had also seen women encircling the Greenham Common airbase, and again, although I hadn't been involved, I heard about it from a cousin of your dad's, who had been there. I wanted to find out more. In Eastbourne and in Hastings I went to a few CND meetings, and at one stage, I arranged for a couple of the Eastbourne people to come and talk to the Hastings group about Non Violent Direct Action. Before becoming pregnant with you, I went on a big CND rally at Easter.

Also, to the - now late - EP Thompson's question, "Gentle Guardian reader, where will you be on October 22nd?" I can give a positive reply. In a hand-embroidered smock, pale green maternity trousers and plimsolls, I, with your dad and your brothers, boarded one of the special CND chartered trains that day, bound for Waterloo. Your dad couldn't do the normal quota of marching which was, for him, synonymous with protest, partly on account of my size and swollen ankles (whose significance will become apparent later) and also because your brothers were too young to walk far anyway. But we fully participated in all the festivities laid on for young children, and came home with balloons and masses of literature. One booklet, in particular, told us that 11% of our electricity bill went to fund the nuclear industry, and proposed a scheme whereby you could withhold that 11% and put it into a special fund. I wish now that I'd looked into that further. Much of the discourse around nuclear power has shifted now, but that still seems worthwhile.

It was also through CND that I found out about the local Greenham Support Group, and that it was there that all my sympathies lay. While men in CND tended to compare the fire power of relative nuclear arsenals, women argued from the emotional imperative that all nuclear weapons, everywhere, were evil. I could channel all my politics, in the true sense of my politics being everything I was, into this movement. This I did, from June onwards. There were no conflicts with motherhood. Most meetings were in the evenings anyway, and many of the other things that needed to be done could be completed when the children were with me. Someone once remarked on how much I got done, when I had two children already and I was pregnant with a third. I didn't point out that it was precisely because I was in that situation, and needed to do other things as well, that so much got done.

Also, most women in the Greenham Support Group had children much older than mine, and had literally outgrown the need for NCT. I found it refreshing, once or twice a week, to be reminded that there were stages of life and of campaigning that did not centre on the bearing of young life, and also to be reminded that a time might come when I too had no need of these support groups. I remember Rosie - Rosie James - most clearly, with her vibrant dark hair, two boys aged four and six and a house which always looked as if she had just moved in. By coincidence, her husband worked, like your dad, in the Unemployment Benefit Office.

It was Rosie who lent me the smock I wore on October 22nd, which she had embroidered in bright colours some years before, when smocks were really trendy. Although that time had now passed, they were still eminently suitable for maternity wear, and I was not the first pregnant friend she lent it to. What I appreciated, though, apart from the kindness, was the amount of knowledge that lay behind Rosie's skill. She knew much of the social history of smocking - who wore what type of smock and when. She also informed me that the green and gold colours which I loved so much were technically wrong, and that the traditional smock would have had white stitching.

I think that that kind of marriage of women's craftwork and knowledge was one of the best things to come out of that phase of the women's movement, and although I see few signs of it around me now, I hope it is not lost. It would have been an invaluable part of anything I might have taught you.

I also especially remember her friend Sue Marriott, who had light brown wild hair, very much the same texture as Jan Moore's, but darker. She also had an equally wild nose, which had been broken in childhood. She too was very practical as well as well-informed, and used to produce lovely tie-dye scarves, with dove motifs, for fund-raising. (I still have one, and often use it as a drape at school.) Intrinsically one of the most gentle of women, she was actually responsible for our group name - Hastings Women for Survival. While most of us wanted to be Women for Peace, Sue maintained that if a soldier came up your street and attacked your children you would fight back, so Survival was more appropriate. She must have argued her case persuasively, for we went for the pragmatic name rather than the idea we actually stood for. I still wonder now if people confused us with mountain rescue squads or lifeboat teams.

So while it was true that most of the women in Hastings Women for Survival were interested in all women's rights, and that would have included choices in childbirth, although that was not their campaigning issue, there was scant interest the other way round. When push came to shove, to choose a surprisingly apt metaphor, NCT women were not, on the whole, fighting for structural change, but for tinkering with the system. Of one woman that I remember, that was not true, at least at that time. An active NCT breastfeeding counsellor, Pam Summerfield was also heavily involved in Women for Survival. Like Sue, physically she reminded me of one of the Lincolnshire Women's Group - Lynne. She had the same fine, dark, flattish hair with wavy edges, and the same silver-framed glasses and bright eyes behind them. Although she didn't come out with Lynne's pertinent phrases there was the same hurt intelligence in her eyes. When my tragedy happened, I was to find out what hers had been.

So, although I remember having young children around as a time I never want to go back to, I had managed to channel my energies into friendships and campaigns that, for their time, I still consider worthwhile, and that I value now, for having had them. Yes, the world has moved on, Louise, and if you could come back now it would not be the same one you left all those years ago, but that does not invalidate what I believed in and what I tried to do. And I do not feel your brothers suffered. Or at least, they would have suffered far more if there had been only me and them.

There is one more person I must introduce to you now, Louise. Kathy Slater was a friend of Tina's - or perhaps I should say special friend, because most people in St. Leonards seemed to be friends of the gregarious Tina. Kathy and Tina had met at a local doctor's surgery and discovered a mutual interest in vegetarianism. Although Kathy was ten years younger than me, her two daughters, Kim and Nel, were exactly the same age as Benjamin and Sam, and her third baby was due a week before you. I also recall knowing at that time, that she had lost a baby at twenty weeks of pregnancy - another daughter. And again, when Tina told me this, I felt a strange unease, which was more than being unsure how to talk to Kathy about it if the subject cropped up. Kathy had thickly cropped dark hair, with matching straight eyebrows, and legs that any non-feminist woman would die for. She complemented them by going bare-legged much of the time. She also had a shy-ish and becoming smile. Most of the time when I saw her it was with Tina, but we were to become acquaintances, if not friends.

Given the general tenor of many of the conversations I had with Tina, and the somewhat esoteric knowledge she often shared with me, it came as little surprise to discover that she was intending to visit the annual Festival of Mind, Body and Spirit in London. I was becoming increasingly interested in pathways and meridians, and when she asked me to come with her, I accepted. She would bring the baby, and both our older boys would spend the Saturday with their dads. I would be exactly seventeen weeks pregnant.

We got a lift with a couple who seemed very normal but were doing some strange psychic research, some of which Tina had typed up to earn some extra money. Of course, when we got there, the Festival was so vast that it was hard for someone inexperienced, and therefore gullible, like me, to separate the genuine, and in many cases, proven, therapies, from the charlatans. It was lack of cash that prevented me making a complete fool of myself, and buying all sorts of rubbish. A little learning is a dangerous thing. I remember some literature that promoted birth control without the aid of any kind of device, operation or medication at all - you simply told yourself you didn't want a baby. It clearly hadn't worked for me recently. Tina seemed very interested in this, so I didn't tell her that my expecting you was a direct result of taking exactly that kind of attitude. Perhaps my karma had not been right. As she now has ten children, I don't know if she ever tried it or not.

I also had my back manipulated for what seemed to me a small fortune, although it was supposedly a discount rate. The manipulator also told me that there was a lot of noise and that she did not really have the time to give me a proper treatment, although I should get some temporary relief. So she had covered herself, and when the pain started again, as it was to a week later, I could not really say that I had wasted my money. And I did enjoy the short session, as peaceful music and incense floated around me. But it was my tummy, rather than my back, which seemed to feel the most relief, and experienced a sort of turning over feeling - not at all unpleasant. Not at all unpleasant, because I realised I was feeling you move, and it was as if you were responding to the treatment. Baby Dominic, normally quite a fractious baby, seemed to have had a good time too, and had slept most of the day, obviously surrounded by positive vibes and goodwill.

It was a warm summer evening as we were driving back. John, the bloke who was driving, asked Tina something in a laid-back way, that I didn't quite understand, as she began to feed the baby. Quite tired by all the day's new experiences, I lay my head against the window and felt myself start to doze off. Again, I felt that fluttering in my tummy that was like a butterfly's wings. "Tina, I've just felt the baby move."

She looked at me in a way I had never before seen her look - the joy was not just for me, but for a new life coming into the world.

"Penny's just felt the baby move," she told the couple in the front. My news was shared with these strangers that I would never see again, but now, we were bound by these special early moments in your life. I was going to have a baby. I was going to have you.

19 The Gift of a Name

...... the truth is that when one woman gives birth to another, to someone who is like her, they are linked together for life in a very special way.

About ten days after my visit to the Festival, I whiled away one lovely summer's afternoon with your brothers at Rosie's house. The kitchen and a living room at the back of the house had at one stage been knocked through, creating a huge white space, and the original wall had been replaced with a rustic-looking breakfast bar. There were bare floorboards in the kitchen area, and a faded oriental carpet covered most of the floor of the sitting-room space. This area also contained a couple of crumpled armchairs, which, like most other things about the house, seemed to have been left accidentally, and would one day be moved to a permanent position. I delighted in this feeling, in Rosie's house, that everything was ephemeral, with a delicious guilty pleasure: it was a place where imposed order ceased to matter, but that was because Rosie thought it unimportant, and had chosen not to control this aspect of her life: she had established different patterns of order, rather as Olivia had, and I loved her for it. I knew that I could never be that free, but I clutched the moments at Rosie's house and, like a child unexpectedly given extra sweets, I hoarded them jealously and later, savoured every one.

This particular afternoon was even more luscious than most. I liked motherhood best when I could spend time thinking of your brothers as little people rather than beings who seemed to exist solely to be my responsibility. I didn't consciously want to unload this weight of responsibility onto someone else, but I didn't want to own it continuously either. That afternoon, at Rosie's house, provided just such a time. White-framed French windows, casually open, led from the sitting room out into Rosie's narrow but long garden. A walled garden, it was safe for your brothers to explore, which they did happily while Rosie and I talked lazily, running in from time to time, just to check I was still there. If motherhood could be always this, I thought - but then, it will be, soon. Again, I felt you move, as white butterflies landed on deep purple Buddleia spears, and my hand moved over my stomach, and Rosie smiled in an indulgent way.

Because of the geography of her house - on a main road between Hastings and St. Leonards, and, even for a non-driver like me, easy to get to; because of her involvement in CND and the women's movement, and because of the relaxed nature of her house and of her personality, Rosie was rarely without visitors. Sue, the woman who was so determined that we should be women for Survival, visited Rosie most days - usually several times. So did Rosie's sister-in-law Miriam, who had given birth to enormous twin boys a year before, and derived a great deal of support from her visits to the house. She also happened to know Tina - but then a lot of people did. Hastings is a surprisingly small place.

In the two-and-a-half hours that I was there, both of these women visited, as did Rosie's next-door neighbour. Julia was, I guessed, like us, in her early thirties. Several years before, Rosie and her husband had decided that they did not need all the space that they had, and had split their house into two, and rented half of it out. Although Julia's half was totally separate, it seemed as though some kind of cord held Rosie and Julia together: it was something different from the bond either of landlady and tenant, or of friendship. Julia, whose smoking - even around the children - chunky jewellery and short skirt suggested brashness, became noticeably softer around Rosie, and also seemed to anticipate Rosie's movements. Rosie would go to collect the washing in, or to put the kettle on, and find that Julia had just done it. Julia's appearance belied what turned out to be a constant preoccupation with psychic interests, confirmed by her comment to Rosie- "You are still the spirit that inhabits my house."

Julia also claimed to be able to see people's auras. While my own interest in psychic matters was developing, largely under Tina's influence, and being sustained by our visit to the Festival, auras seemed inherently uninteresting to me - I still don't really know why. I think Julia claimed to be able to see mine, but I can't now remember what she said. Sitting at the breakfast bar, surrounded by a number of used coffee mugs, I watched your brothers playing near the roots of one of Rosie's two horse chestnut trees. Then I noticed something strangely, but unpleasantly familiar, about the suspicious shape of Sam's shorts. Too busy playing. I went outside, my suspicions confirmed by smelling him. Normally, I would have got upset - not with him, but at the situation. But I still continued to feel relaxed, as I went back into the house. Rosie asked,

"Would you like me to see if I can find some spare pants?"

"Yes please." And while I cleaned him up, I knew that I had been aware that the situation would be handled easily and not even turn into a problem.

Rosie smiled from one of the armchairs as I went back into the sitting room, and Sam resumed his game, watched through the dusty window. The depth of shine in her eyes equalled that on her hair from this slothfully fulfilled sun. I could hear the drone of traffic from the front of the house melded with that of insects at the back. With something of an effort, I tried to pick up the drift of the conversation. It hadn't shifted much from auras, but the wave of discussion was drawing away. Rosie, pragmatic but kind, said,

"Well, I don't claim to have any psychic awareness in any way, shape or form. But I do know that, the first time you see a baby, you know who it is. It looks totally different from how it will grow up, but you still know what its character is going to be, straight away." Rosie, Miriam and I thought of our own children, the momentous hours after birth and what we had learnt then, and we agreed. And I thought of you in that coming time, and the moment when I would know you. "So this is who you are!" Julia, I supposed, knew what each of the children was like from their auras. I also suddenly realised that there were four women and six children in and around the house, yet a summer spell was over it. It was neither crowded nor fractious. Miriam's babies were asleep, each filling his side of the push chair, and Rosie's boys played elsewhere in the garden. Distinguished from the general background hum, a bumble bee buzzed languidly by the French window before dropping onto one of the sunflowers that Rosie had planted next to a south-facing wall.

For a few minutes, we seemed to lapse into a kind of trance. Eventually this was broken by Rosie, who sort of carried on the conversation.

"Julia can always tell the sex of a baby, before it's born. I've known her get thirteen out of thirteen right, in the time I've known her. Do you want to know what she thinks yours is?"

"Yes please." Suddenly I am animated again. I believe in this woman, her gold chain necklace, bracelet and anklet, and her predictions. I believe in her magic - whatever she says, it will be true. She will not just interpret - she will make things happen.

I look across at Julia. I expect her to affirm Rosie's statement - after all, she has a gift. But she looks like I used to at family gatherings when my mother used to make me play the piano to show me off. I feel slightly uncomfortable, and I don't know why. I don't really know what has gone wrong. The living presence of Rosie and Miriam seems to have solidified. They are wax figures in the corner of the room.

"What do you think, then?" I look directly at Julia, and, for a fraction of a second, her narrow yellow eyes meet mine before she looks away again.

"I think it's a girl." She does not say it to me. It is a general comment, directed somewhere at the room. I look round. The other two women come back into focus. Rosie looks thrilled for me, and I know she will feel, as Sylvia felt when Amber was born, that you will be a daughter, not just for me, but a statement for our group. Miriam looks rather pissed off, but smiles bravely. I am thrilled to the womb in which you live, and move, and have your being. I realise I am not surprised by Julia's predictions - she has confirmed what I already know - that at last, my daughter is coming to me. Already, I can separate the words from the way in which she has said them. I cannot understand why there was no note of pleasure in her voice, and why it fell only as a dark thud, without resonance. But it seems totally irrelevant anyway, in the light of what Julia has said. The baby is a girl, or a boy. There is no other possibility. And it is a girl. Nothing else matters, not even the way in which Julia steadfastly continues to avoid my eyes.

"Have you thought of a name for the baby?" asks Miriam. She has dark permed curls framing her face. They are dry and look worn out.

"Rebecca Louise. They've all been going to be called Rebecca, but the other two came out with the wrong bits."

The other women smile, even Julia. The tension is broken. It's a lovely afternoon again - when you feel that you're actually inside the summer, wrapped in it. I elucidate.

"The very first time we ever discussed having children, Paul said that if we had a daughter, Rebecca was a good name, and it's also what I'd had in mind for years - partly because I had a great-grandmother called Rebecca, and I like the idea of carrying on family names. Actually, before Benjamin came along, it was going to be Rebecca Susan, after another great-grandmother, who brought my mum up. Then between having Benjamin and Sam, I changed it - literally out of the blue. Paul's mum asked one day what we were going to call the baby, and on impulse, I said 'Rebecca Louise.' Paul said that was the first he knew about it, but that it was much better. I said it was the first I knew about it too, but it sounded right.

"Isn't it difficult choosing names though?" said Miriam almost inaudibly, as though the task of coming up with Jonathan and Joseph had also worn her out.

"The thing is," intercepted Rosie wisely, "a name is a gift for the recipient, who will have that, even if they never have anything else, for the rest of their life. It's not actually a gift for the giver, although we expect to choose names that give us satisfaction."

"A friend of mine at university" (I said, thinking again of Little Pete) "used to say that your name calls you into being."

"I think that's true," replied Rosie. "It's amazing how unsatisfactory it feels when you know a baby's been born and no-one has given it a name. It's harder to relate to it, somehow."

"And that's the first thing they do with foundling children, isn't it," added Miriam. On the news, they always say, 'The baby has been named Geoffrey, or Agnes, after the person who found them.'"

"Or Holly, or Noel, if it's around Christmas." Julia had re-joined the conversation.

"So it's definitely Rebecca?" Rosie wanted to make sure.

"Yes. I've tried changing it several times in my head, but nothing else seems right. The nearest I came was Anna Rebecca. I thought that had a nice ring to it" - approval from the other women - "but then I realised the initials were ARS, so that made it a non-starter."

We shared the joke of the impending catastrophe from which I had rescued this unborn child, then your brothers came in from the garden. It was nearly time to go. Rosie's house was on your dad's route from work, so he would pick us up. But he did not like hanging around - he wanted to arrive and depart straight away. So I heavily rose from the breakfast bar, inevitably put several of the coffee cups in the sink, and started collecting together all the belongings that

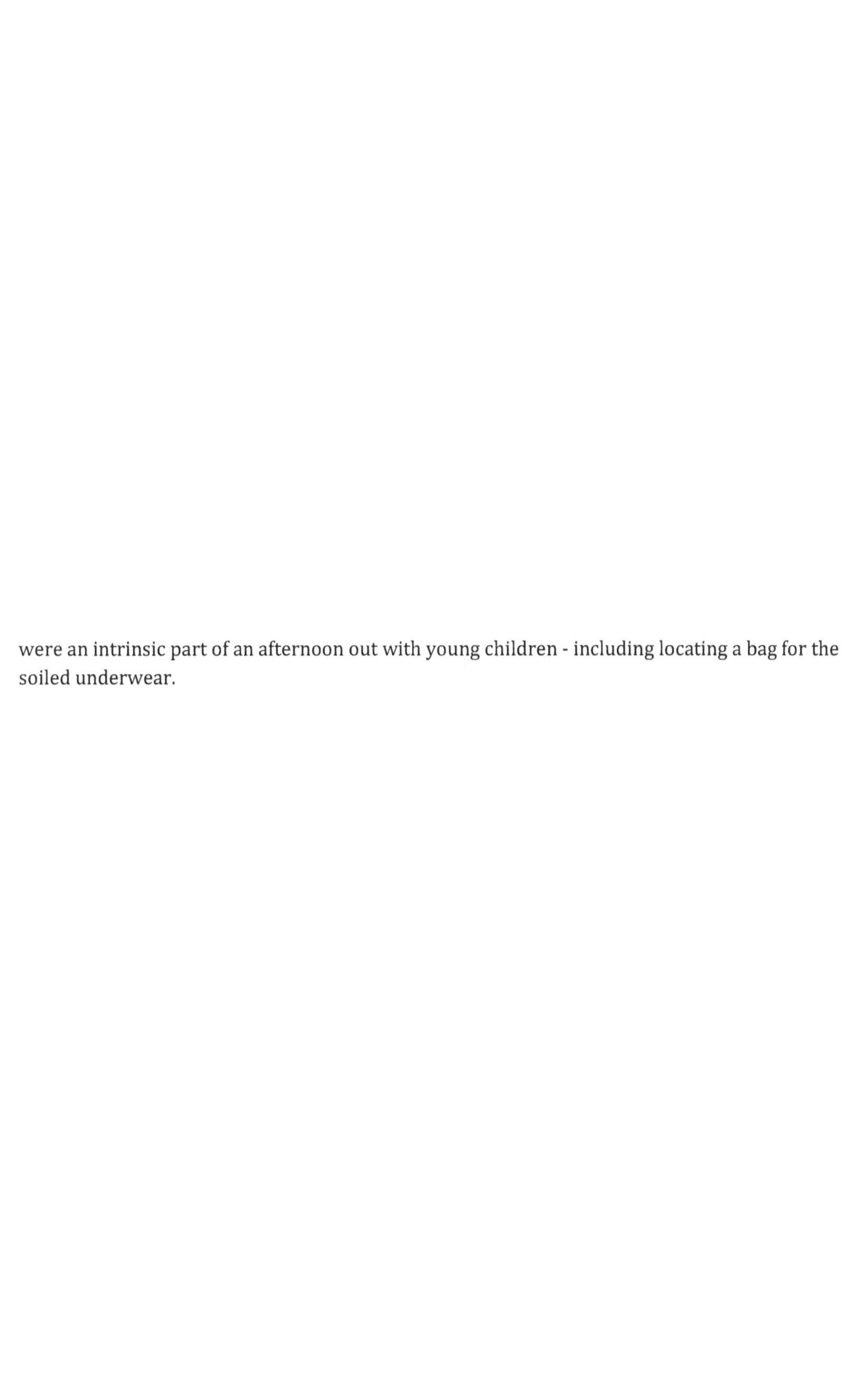

were an intrinsic part of an afternoon out with young children - including locating a bag for the soiled underwear.

Part Three

Late Pregnancy

It is only by putting it into words that I make it whole; this wholeness means that it has lost the power to hurt me; it gives me, perhaps because by doing so I take away the pain, a great delight to put the severed parts together. Perhaps this is the strongest pleasure known to me... we – I mean all human beings - are connected with this; we are the words; we are the music; we are the thing itself.

> *Only by the form, the pattern,*
> *Can words or music reach*
> *The stillness, as a Chinese jar still*
> *Moves perpetually in its stillness.*

When my life should have been at its most holistic, it was, in fact, at its most fragmented. In Lincolnshire, I was my family, the house and the land, and later, some other women, yet virtually from the time of Sam's birth onwards, I had stood frozen in that wood, fearing to make decisions which would cut me off forever from all other possibilities, yet neurotically impelled to make precisely those decisions, to make them irrevocably. By contrast, as the autumn of 1983 approached, and with it my own ripeness, I was, ostensibly, involved in several disparate things, but for me, they were folding together into a seamless garment.

You know already about the NCT and how important it was in representing the chance to have you the way I believed babies should be born. I began classes with Jayne about ten weeks before you were due, and it was her first full set of classes since she'd qualified. Since our first awkward meeting, I had got to know a lot more about the woman behind the big house, the expensive clothes and the tragedy. She was well-organised, caring, knowledgeable, and very funny. We could now talk easily about anything, including the twins, though this is probably more of a testament to her humanity and courage than anything to do with me. Nevertheless, I never forgot that she was someone not to be trifled with, and a story I heard of her imperiously, rather than apologetically, sending back food in an expensive restaurant, came as no surprise.

I think that most of the women at those classes, to some extent or other, knew Jayne, the breastfeeding counsellor Pam, and one or two other people, before we even started. We also knew that we could go on knowing these people after we had had our babies - that they would not disappear out of our lives forever. Even on its own, that provided a more relaxed atmosphere than the hospital ever had. There was also a conscious acknowledgement that relaxation was something to be provided before being taught and practised, rather than something which we, as individuals, had to attempt to achieve under somewhat trying circumstances.

It seems axiomatic now that, if you know what is happening to your body, you will be less afraid when the pain starts, but when I started NCT classes I was amazed at how little I had known when your brothers were born. I drank in all the information about me and you that Jayne could provide, from a well of the purest water. I'm glad I did. You deserve no less.

But it was the ambience of the classes that made them so special, rather than simply the quality of information. I enjoyed the intimacy of being in someone else's home, rather than in an impersonal hospital room, for a couple of hours a week. I liked being given coffee in one of Jayne's mugs, rather than a sterile plastic cup. Jayne, who had a good eye for interior design, had made the room extremely comfortable; not only with the obligatory cushions, but with soft lighting that cast gentle shadows over the sage greens, browns and faded blues of her furnishings. She used a lot of visualisation in the relaxation techniques we learned, including holding our babies after delivery, and focusing on the momentous nature of birth, rather than the pain itself. And although it was to be so utterly different for you and me, and your dad, I still have those moments, and they cannot be taken from me. I remember waking up one morning after one of the classes. Before I was properly conscious, and my eyes were still glued with sleep, I could feel you in bed beside me, no longer in my womb, and I reached out and cuddled you for a long time before allowing myself to wake up.

Pam Summerfield, whom I knew already from my Hastings Women for Survival involvement, was to be the breastfeeding counsellor for our group. She had been a breastfeeding counsellor for a long time, and she did it well, although she was talking of giving it up in the near future. Her daughter Heather was now six, and Pam did not intend having any more children. Another very active woman, she now wanted to become more involved in other projects she had started to give her time to, like setting up a wholefood co-op. On the verge of being able to run with the idea that there was another world that did not involve pregnancy and childbirth, she was ready to move on. But she was prepared to give her time and experience until new counsellors were trained.

Pam sat in at most of the classes, usually as a silent observer. Most of what directly and immediately concerned us was the delivery. But at one stage she gave a talk. Like Jayne, she had a good way of talking to a group, providing information yet giving her audience respect. Her voice was softer than Jayne's and surprisingly deep. She explained to us about the anatomy of the breast, how milk was produced, how to "plug in" the baby and told us to feed on demand. She gave us the latest information on how a baby recognises its own mother's breast, the sucking reflex, and the importance of suckling within the first half hour of birth. She also competently answered any questions that came to mind at the time.

It was during the talk that some of us became aware of one woman who seemed uncomfortable. Jenny was sitting opposite me, and although the light was not harsh I could see that she was very flushed, and was shifting on her cushion as though desperate for the toilet - a condition we could all identify with. Someone leaned over and asked if she was all right. She said she was, and Pam's talk carried on.

I didn't know much about Jenny. We'd not had that many classes, and partners had come to a couple of them, which tended to put a damper on the women getting together for a chat. The men tended to sit around awkwardly. unable to share the pregnancy with other men in the way that the women could. When the men weren't there, we tended, during breaks, to chat for a few minutes before moving on to another member of the group - rather like a party. We were all in this together, and we did not favour special friendships. Jenny was a bit taller than me - about five foot six - with pale skin and rather greasy henna-red curls that she scraped back. Her Swedish husband was called Bjorn, and although she had taken his family name on marriage, she had kept hers too, so she was on Jayne's register as Jennifer Cole Andersen. I also knew that, like me, she had been a teacher, and was planning to return after maternity leave - something still fairly unusual, even so short a time ago.

After Pam's talk had finished, and we'd had our coffee, Jenny seemed more relaxed. It was when we had questions that what had really been troubling her emerged. Jenny did not like having her nipples touched - not by Bjorn, not by anyone. She couldn't even bear to touch them herself, it made her feel so dysfunctional. She wanted to breastfeed her baby, but just didn't think she'd be able to, and if she couldn't, she would feel that she had failed. I simply wanted to tell her to pull herself together and to get on with feeding the baby when it arrived. Pam, needless to say, was a good deal more sympathetic and promised to give Jenny all the support she could, when the time came. Sadly, both Jenny and I were to add to the sum of Pam's experience as a breastfeeding counsellor, but not in ways that either of us, at that stage, could have anticipated.

Of us all, it was Jenny who seemed the most uncertain about the birth. She asked the most questions about what the pains were like, how long each sort of pain was likely to last, and, it seemed that she was always asking about the breathing.

"So when do I do the shallow breathing? Is this O.K?" And she would go into a demonstration.

"So when do I do the heavy breathing?" Another demonstration. Jenny's questions about her breathing came to be something of a standing joke - which she readily joined in with. Again, to my shame, I was somewhat irked and impatient about this, although I tried not to be, since I knew I'd had the benefit of two previous deliveries. But, although the other women in the group were kinder than I was - or at least, more tolerant - I know they would all have agreed that the one least likely to show courage in the face of great pain was Jenny. How wrong we were.

One of the things we had to do, on the evenings our partners weren't there, was to massage someone else. This too added to our feeling of a shared experience. That was how I met Beth Marshall.

Beth was expecting her second child. Her first, a daughter, Isla, was two. It was difficult to tell in an advanced stage of pregnancy, but I thought Beth had probably had a rounded figure before she became pregnant this time. She wore glasses - trendy ones, with small metal frames, but her eyes still looked vaguely into the middle distance, as if they could not quite make things out, but had given up trying. She had sleek hair, cut short in interesting angles at the sides, and its plum colour had a glossy uniformity to it that suggested it was not the colour she had started out with. Beth wore the kind of ethnic Indian dresses that I myself favoured. I happened to catch a glance at Jayne's register as I began to massage Beth's well-covered shoulders, and was delighted to discover that she lived just up the road from me - in St. Andrew's Road, right by the church. I was then astonished to discover that, when her baby came, she would be thirty-eight. I had taken her for my age, or younger.

She had the voice of a dove landing. Her shoulders, heavy from stress and carrying a two-year old, eventually smoothed themselves out, and I saw her eyes close. By the time we changed over, I knew that I wanted to know far more about this woman with the soft body, soft dresses and soft voice. And I knew that, whatever I did find out, it would not disappoint.

So my involvement with the NCT became a good deal more than measuring out my life with coffee mornings. I was learning how to have a baby properly - I was preparing for you.

By the time the ante-natal course started, I had already embarked on another project that reminded me I could still do things that used my mind to good effect. In September I had enrolled on a daytime course, run through the WEA, and aimed at women. A similar course had run the previous year, and many of the same women were, apparently, on this one. The lecturer, Judy Lawson, taught at the University of Sussex, and it was brilliant to have this tentative link again with my undergraduate days. So, on Thursday mornings, plied with anything your brothers could conceivably want during the course of a morning out, we set off intrepidly for the Labour Party rooms - situated in the same Regency Square as Dr Walker's surgery. In one of the square, wood-panelled and lino rooms I did the course while they played, either at my feet or with the other women's children.

I remember one particularly vivid discussion when we were talking about maternal love. The woman who had given the paper maintained that there is something genetic in this love -

that we love our children because they are ours. I knew that Judy and I had had similar difficulties with our children when she said that this was not the case, and that a number of women did not love their children automatically, that they had to learn to love them, and that also, their children came to them as complete strangers and it was only through looking after them and spending time with them that such love developed. And that the obverse was true. Mothers could equally love adopted children as if they were their own. She asserted that the idea of a genetic maternal love was, to some degree, a social construction, reminding women that their reason for being and the skills that they "naturally" developed were all connected with reproduction. In Judy's scenario, therefore, women who fell in love with their babies did so because of who those children were rather than what they represented. This made that love more, rather than less, valid.

I had never thought of it like that before. You, Louise, were the one I expected to give instinctive, maternal, love to, because I thought you were going to be me, and that I would love you, not as I loved myself, but as I wished I loved myself, and as I wished I had been loved. And while that did not change, I began to have more respect for the kind of love I had for your brothers.

The actual title of the course was Women in Other Cultures, which more "intellectual" establishments would not, at that stage, touch with a barge pole, on the understanding that white women studying black women in detail is wrong. Until there are more black women in our higher education establishments, they argue, white women can teach only from a position of relative power, and that is unethical. However, I was totally unaware of this argument when I did the course, and it provided insight into a whole new world for me, particularly through the writings of Buchi Emecheta. It will probably come as no surprise to you to know that I wrote my first paper for the group about childbirth in other cultures. I remember reading it to the group one sunny Thursday morning. I knew it was a well-researched paper, and I gained enormous satisfaction from doing it. I was gratified too, that it generated some good discussion. The development of my family and of my own education no longer seemed so desperately incompatible: I felt sure, that, when you arrived, there would still be time for both. It was in a truly bizarre way that that time was found.

21 Misgivings

I said to my soul, be still and wait without hope
For hope would be hope for the wrong thing; wait without love
For love would be love of the wrong thing; there is faith
But the faith and the love and the hope are all in the waiting.

When I was about thirty-three weeks pregnant, I took your brothers to Hove one Sunday, to see Lesley, Ian and their daughters. Your dad had some work to do at his office, and although I was now more comfortable with him going away overnight, I hated being alone with the children at weekends, when just about every mother I knew had a husband at home. We went by train, and this made me feel quite adventurous.

Lesley and Ian were happily settled in their spacious, yet unprepossessing, new home. It was an inter-war semi, full of bay windows and stained glass in the fanlights. It had a patio and garden, substantial but not large. The road - or avenue - was wide, but nowhere near the boulevard scale of many of the roads in Hove. It occurred to me that, in paying three times for their house what we had paid for our flat, they were buying into an area: ironically, our flat, with its huge rooms, had the same amount of living space - albeit one less bedroom - was on the same kind of wide road and had the same proximity to the sea. Nevertheless, we were relatively so poor, and they were relatively so wealthy, that I drank in every feature almost with awe but also rather guiltily, as if I was not sure if we actually had a right to be there. Lesley and Ian certainly had not been attracted by the house's decorations and features, and were in the middle of ripping many of them out, and, in many ways making their new house look as like the old one as they could.

I sat around for a lot of the day. A salty grey wind blew up the road and brought a mist with it. Benjamin and Sam were quite content playing with the different toys on offer to them, and Lesley got them drinks, so they did not demand a lot of my attention. There was some niggling between Lesley's youngest and her two older daughters, but I felt that it could easily be handled, and as I folded my arms over my enlarged abdomen, I thought in contented terms about the coming future. Only one thing rather niggled at me. Although I had hardly been on my feet, my ankles had swollen substantially by the time we left, and now, this was happening most days. In fact, my ankles were slightly puffy even when I got up in the mornings. But I told myself this was simply a feature of this pregnancy. As I later reflected, while not the happiest day, it was the last one before I was to begin to feel the walls of my life closing in on me.

The following day, I breezed into my ante-natal appointment. At the previous one, Dr Walker had said that I had a big baby in there, that I could stop taking the iron tablets which had been disagreeing with me, and that everything was fine - so good, in fact, that I did not have to go back for three weeks.

And if pride does come before a fall, then I had more than my fair share of warnings. A couple of weeks before, I had been shopping in the St. Leonards Boots one morning when I met Kathy, Tina's vegetarian friend. Whereas your brothers were at playschool so I had a little time to myself, Kathy was surrounded by her family, and her husband Robbin stopped Kim and Nel sabotaging the shop while she and I had a chat. (This was quite genial of him, since at the time he was an active animal rights campaigner targeting pharmaceutical companies.)

In many ways, when I look back, I don't like the person I was then. Kathy asked very politely how the pregnancy was going, so of course I jumped in with over-the-top enthusiasm, and I can imagine everyone in the shop could hear me. Eventually, when I had got to the end of my spiel, I remembered to ask Kathy how she was getting on.

"It's rather a small baby," she answered quietly. "and they have to do another scan. They're not sure if it's growing all right."

Again, I know that I made the right sounds, reassuring her. What I could not know, at that time, was how much the loss of one baby could inform the next pregnancy. I could understand Kathy being worried - I could not know that she would be sick to her soul with it. And to my shame, I know I felt in some way proud, that I was doing better. Feelings like that are not concealed simply by the absence of articulating them.

I had also experienced a similar feeling of smug complacency a couple of days later. Again, I was in St. Leonards - walking down St. John's Road, to be precise - when I met Alison, from the toddler group. I can't remember why I was alone. I think your dad must have had an early afternoon and was looking after your brothers while I did some shopping.

The afternoon was gritty and grey, as if it had been badly washed. Alison's eyes looked more faded than ever, and even the putative redness of their lids, caused by the bitter wind, was a bloodless pink. She held out two white paper bags, branded with the Boots logo. Both she and Michael had needed prescriptions and the cost had absorbed most of the money they had to live on for the week.

"It's probably as well I'm not pregnant, if I've got to take these. But I'd rather be pregnant and not be able to take the tablets. We've been trying since May and nothing's happened yet."

"Maybe after Christmas, when the year's turned," I replied. I wasn't really sure why I said that, other than to alleviate Alison's obvious despondency. On one level I did feel sorry for her plight and it was something positive to say: on another, I felt superior. I could create babies whenever I chose - big babies, with no complications. I don't remember, but I probably gave Alison the rundown of exactly how well my pregnancy was going, if not at that meeting, at a toddler group session. Mrs. Sensitive told her exactly what she wanted to hear.

But it was also at this time that something happened that will make me question forever my part in the universe and why you, and I, were put on this world. At the time, I took little notice at a conscious level, and yet, when it mattered, I found out that I had absorbed every detail. For it was at the end of October (I think) that an Esther Rantzen programme went out called "The Lost Babies." It told me that the parents who grieved most desperately for their dead babies were parents who had not seen or cuddled their little ones at all, those babies having been "lost" as a misguided act of kindness. It also told me about a medical condition I had never heard of before, and which only people in the medical profession seem to know about. It is called anencephaly. It is related to spina bifida and hydrocephalus, but unlike them, any child affected by it has no chance whatsoever of surviving. The baby has no skull and only a rudimentary brain. One baby in the programme with this condition had lived for nearly a week. Her parents had known there was no hope, but they had spent all the time with their daughter that they could. Psychologically, they had survived a lot better than other parents whose babies had simply been taken away.

Looking at the programme, I could understand why it had seemed the kindest thing to take away an anencephalic baby. The only pictures of them are in books, and they do not look pretty. They have faces but that's it. There is no head above the eyebrows. And because they cannot digest the liquor they have floated in before birth, their faces, and particularly their eyes, take on a bloated appearance. And of course, such babies are known only by their medical condition. Lumped together and given a label, they are all the same.

I remember waking up that night, as I felt you move near my ribcage, with that horrendous image of an anencephalic baby in my mind. A part of me, I knew, related to what I had seen, but another part dismissed it. Even I could see that to worry about my unborn child having a condition of which I had never heard before, and had discovered about by accident, was absurd.

So, as I have said, it was with a light step and a feeling of nonchalance that I attended my thirty-three week ante-natal check-up. It may be a good thing that I had those three weeks of complete faith in the normality of the pregnancy, even if I was particularly unfeeling, since, from that appointment onwards, things were never to be the same again. I went in, bloated in body as well as in mind. When I came out, I looked the same, but a pin had been taken to my mental state and it was slowly deflating.

The first problem seemed relatively straightforward, certainly in the light of what was to happen, but it caused anxiety at the time. After he had examined me, Dr Walker checked my ankles. If anything, they were more swollen than they had been the previous day, at Lesley's house. He told me to rest, which of course I regarded as something of a joke, and told him so. He became a mite sterner.

"You must. Oedema can lead to problems."

"Right." Suitably chastised, I remained silent.

"I'm also making a note about the amount of liquor you're carrying." (He pronounced it with a long 'I' sound.) "You seem to have rather a lot."

"That's not unusual for me," I replied, feeling that I was reassuring him. "I carried a lot of water with my previous two babies." This was indeed true. I was not clutching at straws. Both my previous labours had been signalled by a breaking of waters sufficient to drown a small village.

I think your dad must have been looking after your brothers that afternoon, following his weekend's overtime. I remember that, when I came out of the surgery I was on my own, and that I didn't want to go straight home. I could have kicked myself for not asking what sort of problems oedema could lead to, but at least I knew that I could find out. What disturbed me was that this was the first time that anything had ever gone wrong in one of my pregnancies, and I felt a general unease which extended much further than concern about swollen ankles. I decided to go for a coffee, and, if the truth be told, probably a cream cake. I'd always used pregnancy as an excuse for a bit of a pig out, reckoning that if I was going to lose my figure anyway, I might as well do it in style. Something that might have puzzled me, if I had thought about it, was that I had only put on just over a stone in weight: I didn't think I was eating less than I had when I was expecting your brothers, but with them, I'd been well on the way to three stone by now. I simply thought that this time, I must be doing it right - just putting on the amount of weight that the medical profession thought I should.

It was another dismal afternoon, as it had been the day before, and just as it had been when I met Alison. That early winter seemed to specialise in them. I went to the new Debenhams restaurant, improbably renamed Springles, and decorated in green. The staff wore co-ordinating green uniforms, with a flower pattern on the tabard. If I did buy a cake, I gained little pleasure from eating it. Normally I liked it there because, being one floor up, it overlooked the sea, but today the sea was too steely, too restless, too high - as high as I was, looking out, confused. Like me, the Channel was too full of salty water.

I spent one night ostensibly worrying about the oedema. That, at least, was a definite worry. What I could not get away from was this feeling of unease I had felt when I left the doctor's, and which seemed to be gaining momentum, encircling me. At its edges, it was far more than unease. It was a feeling that my life, in a profound, if not literal sense, was to be taken from me and that I had no control in the face of it. In both a consciously and unconsciously inarticulate way I knew that it had something to do with how I felt when I'd seen Esther Rantzen's programme, and something else I was coming to feel more and more - that despite all the evidence to the contrary, I was not going to have a baby.

Yet I never felt worried. Partly this was because, as I have answered people subsequently when they have asked if I suspected anything was wrong,

"I knew, yes, but I didn't want to know."

Other than this "feeling," there was no actual evidence that things were other than within normal parameters - even the problems that were soon to surface. Also, at whatever deep level I knew something was wrong, I also knew that there was nothing I could do. If you worry about the worst, you also hope for the best. It is a kind of superstition. Something told me that all I could do was submit. It is ironic that, throughout my previous two pregnancies, I worried constantly about whether the baby would be all right. With you - never - at least, not consciously.

But the oedema, at least, was a tangible worry, and I also believed at that stage that, if my mind could be put at rest over that, this feeling of unease would leave me - after all, it was Dr Walker's concern about it that had been one of the trigger points. So early the next morning, I rang Jayne.

"Hi, Jayne," I said brightly, "what can you tell me about oedema?"

"Why?" she replied suspiciously.

"Because I've got it, and Simon" - between us, we called Dr Walker by his first name - "said it could lead to problems. But he didn't say what they are. And like a fool, I didn't ask. I didn't think I needed to know until I got outside."

"And like a fool, you've worried about it all night." I could visualise her dimpled smile. She took a big breath, while her brain sorted out what she needed to remember, then continued.

"Well, oedema itself is nothing. Absolutely nothing. But it is uncomfortable. Where it's serious is when it's one of the signs of pre-eclampsia, and of course, no-one wants you having a pre-eclamptic fit. The others, as you probably know, are high blood pressure and proteins in your water. Two of those and you're in trouble. Three and of course you've hit the jackpot. But oedema on its own is nothing. What does he say you've to do? Take it easy?"

"Yes."

Jayne chuckled. I was already feeling loads better.

"Well, it's not easy. You'll just have to persuade that husband of yours to do as much as he can, and you can get the boys organised so that you can put your feet up."

"Yes. I've already made up a three litre bottle of diluted squash, which I can dispense from the settee. There's getting them to the toilet, but there's not a lot I can do about that. We'll have to play quiet indoor games. Simon also told me not to worry."

She chuckled. "Didn't work though, did it?"

"Nope," I concluded, smiling.

"I don't think Simon can have much quarrel with what you're doing. Good luck. I'll see if I can get some people to call on you."

Jayne did that, and with her network we had a steady stream of visitors, many of whom I'd met only once or twice before. Also, your dad did loads of the work, and seemed to be pleased to do it now, on account of the pregnancy.

In a few days, my puffy ankles were nearly back to normal, and my belief that this strange feeling of losing control would also swirl away from my feet, once I'd been reassured about the oedema, was almost borne out. I finished buying all the things I needed for the home delivery, including the copious amounts of brown paper required. But the feeling of my life closing in around me never completely lifted, and some time before my next ante-natal appointment, I realised that, for a few weeks at least, I had deliberately crossed the street whenever I saw a disabled child. I was sickened by my own behaviour, and sickened more by the force that made me do it.

Wait without thought, for you are not ready for thought:
So the darkness shall be the light, and the stillness the dancing. Whisper of running
streams, and winter lightning.
The wild thyme unseen and the wild strawberry,
The laughter in the garden, echoed ecstasy
Not lost, but requiring, pointing to the agony
Of death and birth.

The following Monday, and with renewed hope in view of my reduced ankles, I went for my next ante-natal check. There was to be no let-up in Dr Walker's concern, though. This time, he wrote starkly on my card - "Excess liquor - difficult to feel foetal head." I had a little joke to myself when he wrote that - "I suppose it's got one." The idea of a headless baby seemed too bizarre even to bring to consciousness, inconceivable even as a sick joke.

It was the same scenario the following week, and presumably would have been the same the week after that, only this time, I didn't make it. No, it wasn't premature labour, although at the time, it felt like it. In picking Sam up awkwardly one afternoon, I inflamed a fibroid. I was thirty-six weeks pregnant. We had visitors for the weekend. More friends of your dad's than mine, we had been to their wedding in 1978 - the same year as our own. I didn't know them well, and felt a fool spending their visit time doubled up in bed.

Dr Walker seemed not to mind being called out on a Sunday. I remember his icy hands on my tummy, and again, the recommendation for rest for at least the next few days. He gave me some homoeopathic powders for the inflammation, and they worked. As far as I am aware, this was the first time I had tried a homoeopathic remedy.

But what was really worrying him could be treated neither by his allopathic nor alternative remedies. While I was ill I had three ante-natal visits, two from him and one from Sister Lennox. Not only, he said, could he not feel the baby's head clearly, but what he could feel indicated that it was lying breech. Sister Lennox, who also complained about the amount of amniotic fluid, seemed to be able to feel more accurately than him, and showed me exactly where she thought the baby was lying - with its head up in my ribcage. In that case, I thought, it's the baby's little arms I can feel against me, not her feet. You still weren't very active, but like a lot of babies, you seemed to kick quite a bit of an evening.

It was on the second of his home visits, and as he was putting his stethoscope away that, avoiding eye contact, Dr Walker asked stiffly, "How would you feel about not having this baby at home?"

"Okay" I lied. My stomach lurched. I was gutted. But I did not want him to think that I was putting the health of my baby second to the place of delivery. Getting you born was the main thing, and I knew that your dad was right when he said,

"It doesn't matter how the baby comes out - as long as it does."

But I couldn't explain, either to him or to the doctor that for me, you were part of a whole package of identity and belief around having a baby. That for all the time I had thought about having you, it was always at home, with as little medical interference as possible. I had tried to strike a blow for the right of women to have their babies how they wanted, and now, not only was the medical profession coming in to "rescue" me if I needed it, but it was taking part of me with it.

I grabbed at one final hope.

"If it's breech, can't you turn it?" I remembered a graphic description Tina had given me once, of her doctor turning Dominic, who was in a breech position, at about a similar stage of pregnancy to where I was now. She had been very sick afterwards, but it had worked, and he had been delivered normally.

"There's too much fluid." He hardly seemed to move his lips as he spoke. "Even if I could turn it, I doubt if it would stay there." He left quickly, still avoiding my eyes, obviously not wanting to let me down again if I came up with any more ill-informed suggestions.

Before anything could be decided, Dr Walker said I would need a scan. At least that way we would know for certain which way the baby was lying. Over the next week, I looked up all the information I could find on breech deliveries.

Monday 12th December was marked out as a busy day for me. It was the Meet-A-Mum Christmas party in, of all things, the morning, because that was when we usually met now, and your dad was to take your brothers. Tina had said she'd keep an eye on things at the party. Meanwhile, I was due at the hospital on behalf of the NCT, and then it was my ante-natal that afternoon.

As the local branch of the NCT, we had been negotiating with the hospital to let one of us attend their ante-natal sessions and let parents know of our existence, at least with regard to post-natal support. I had been chosen because I was fairly new, and therefore stood the most chance of negotiating the formidable Sister Neep. It seemed that various members of our branch had had "run-ins" with her over the years. Ostensibly friendly and helpful, once pushed for a commitment, she took the view that "her" mothers were not to be frightened by the idea that, following birth, anything less than perfection was to be expected. Although she had never actually said so, it appeared that she took a dim view of amateur organisations - even well-informed ones - interfering with the work of the hospital. However, since most of the staff had a high regard for what we did, she had to tread carefully. If I could not get her to agree to let us talk to the parents, I was at least to ask to be allowed to distribute our literature.

Sister Neep appeared, at the outset, accommodating enough, as I had been primed. She exuded an air of caring competence, yet tinged with a neurosis in common with women who take on too much and need it all to be done perfectly, living on the edge of deadlines. The muscles round her mouth were tense. And on each side of her face, a line moving up from her mouth had met one coming down from her eyes, and they had joined, bisecting each cheek. In the stark flourescent lighting I could see the dust of face powder nestling in each line.

The outcome was what might have been expected. As Pam, to whom Sister Neep seemed to have taken an irrational dislike, commented, beneath that friendly exterior, there was, indeed, a bitch. Although she ostensibly went along with everything I was saying, she wanted a very tight rein kept on the practicalities. She wanted

a)to make sure I was one of the people who did the talk (since I had yet to quarrel with her),

b) a transcript of what we would say, and

c) advance copies of our literature and our rota. That way, she would be able to "vet" our speakers.

I agreed, thinking that, since we had quite a few new members, it would be fairly easy to set up a new rota of people fresh to the hospital. We had to work within the confines of what she suggested anyway. Of course, what she realised was that it was the people she already knew - and did not want to be let loose on "her" women - who were the real backbone of the NCT.

There were few members with my degree of commitment who would turn out on winter evenings. I did the talk a few times, then even I found that I had better things to do.

Yet, although she was forbidding, there was something about Sister Neep that invited confidence. Because I was heavily pregnant myself, she seemed to regard me as one of "her" mums, even though I had chosen to go outside the hospital system. We started talking about the pregnancy and when the baby was due, and the fact that I would be having a scan, and I might need the hospital services yet. And then I heard myself blurt out, in a flood of honesty,

"I've wanted this baby for so long." Sister Neep looked puzzled. The hue of the powder in those creases seemed to darken. She knew I had two children, and that they weren't very old. "Did you have trouble conceiving then?" she asked candidly.

"No, it's not that. I just have." That would have to do. Never could I explain the torment of that year before your conception, of the mental and emotional journeys I had made. Never could she understand the swing of the pendulum. But what I realised, when stating that sentence, was that at long, long last it was nearly over, that what I had waited for forever was about to come to me. All I had to do was hold out my hand - touch your living flesh. I could so very nearly reach it.

"Let's hope everything goes well then," she wished. There was doubt in her voice, which I did not understand.

That afternoon, I went to my ante-natal appointment. I was thirty-seven weeks pregnant. There was little new that Dr Walker could add. There was still excess liquor, the baby's head could not be felt, and he thought it was probably still breech. He said that he'd written to the consultant gynaecologist, but so far, had received no reply. He contacted the hospital there and then. I was to have the scan at three o'clock the following afternoon - Tuesday, 13th December. I was to see the consultant at four. For the first time since all this concern had started, I wanted to make something of a joke, even if he failed to see the funny side of it.

"I don't know," I said, "where we lived before there was no chance of a home delivery. Now I move to another part of the country, get it all sorted out - and then the baby messes it up for me."

To give him his due, he did smile, and looked straight at me.

"Yes," he said, "trust the baby to mess it up." He smiled again, and he seemed more confident now that something was being sorted out.

As I left the surgery for the last time in that pregnancy, it seemed that, as far as we were all concerned, there were only two possible outcomes. Either you were breech, in which case I would need to have you in hospital, or you weren't - and then I could at least find out what use all that brown paper would be put to.

I don't think that I can take it
'Cos it took so long to bake it
and I'll never have that recipe again.

The Thursday mornings course had not simply made me feel that it was possible both to have a family and to use my mind: it had reawakened my dormant desire to become reacquainted with academic life. I had decided to leave it nine years before, during my MA at Lancaster, when I felt that, for that period in my life, it had nothing left to offer me. I had been told that, once out, you never got back in, but that, of itself, didn't seem sufficient reason to stay. So at the time, I did something I felt would be more rewarding and socially useful, and, much to my mother's perturbation - she thought I was underachieving - went into teaching.

Now, with the research I had been doing for the Women's Group, the NCT, Women for Survival and the Thursday morning group as a platform, I felt ready to renew links with an academic institution, and Sussex University, where I had done my first degree and which one of my friends had once described as my Alma Mater, was offering the perfect course - Women and Education. It was an MA, and although I already had one, I could see it as a stepping-stone to further academic work. It was a part-time course, so I would be able to combine it with looking after you and your brothers. And like the decision to have you, it reflected a perceived expansion of options that was, to a large extent, the result of Tina's influence. Within the tortuous dialogue of whether to have another baby or write, there had existed a sub-text: if I became a writer, would I write fiction or research? Each contained, for me, its own distinct truth, but I felt that, whichever I chose to write would construct my identity as a writer, and I wanted that identity established in my head too, even if there were no chance of my getting a word published.

Then one day, when I was about five months pregnant with you, and Tina and I sat in her front room drinking coffee, I articulated this thought. The sun made oblongs of honey sunlight on the grey wallpaper. I felt the customary tightness in my voice of unmade decision. Tina did not see the remotest problem. She merely said,

"Why not do both?" She asked it in a naive tone, her cheeks glowing, her blue eyes searching me directly.

"Why not do both?" The question lives now, in my mind, as you do. Why choose anything at all, unless you have to? This particular question had hung over me for far longer than whether to have another baby - it was even a conscious echo of being forced to choose, at seventeen, whether to read English at university or History. And when at university, and receiving some form of counselling because of - believe it or not - an identity crisis - I had been advised to take decisions as I came to them. And as that transparent moment of awareness in my Lincolnshire garden, a year before, had shown me, I had done that, and the changes that I had so far made could inform the future. But such moments of illumination were not part of my daily consciousness. The meaning of my being was still a bone that I constantly gnawed away at, believing still, as Sylvia did, that if I did not define myself, somehow my life would be wasted, that I would do - to use her words- "neither what I should have done nor could have done."

Now Tina, her eyes lit like her window through which the sun shone, was showing me, in the innocence of her question, that keeping options open is not a recipe for muddling through or a substitute for clarity of purpose, but a means of owning an excitement of possibilities - like the way Monet painted water. I felt a weight rise from my chest, and changed my position in the slightly shabby armchair so that the dusty light flooded my hair and face and shoulders. Why not do both? Why not do it all?

In my mid-forties, of course, I understand why I couldn't do it all - simply in daily living, you have to make decisions that cut you off from another path. But what I understand now is that what seem to be decisions, in the sense of something that changes the pattern of our life forever, are often not our decisions at all, but a way of having to act because we had no choice. Ultimately it's about personal survival, and that is where we find ourselves, starkly and often surprised by what we have done, for most of us don't know our true selves very well. That is the place where we can start defining our true being, but it is organic, like DNA, and we can start only from the inside and work out. As I was about to discover, forcing a decision will not work - one trauma and it will tumble, leaving you to question all you ever thought you were, or hoped to achieve.

So, somewhat appropriately, I was to go to Sussex University for an interview for an MA in Women and Education on the same day that I was booked into Dexter Hospital for my scan.

Tina rang me on the morning of the interview, to wish me well and to warn me of the icy pavements. The warning was well taken - the corner of Chapel Park Road, where we lived, and St. John's Road, a steep hill which led to the station, was treacherous in cold weather. At the side of the pavement, leading in both directions from the corner, was some wire fencing, like that used in playgrounds, that demarcated the boundary of British Rail land. It was to this that I clung, vastly pregnant, taking mincing steps as the mesh cut into my gloved fingers. I sweated in the pallid sunshine. A few other pedestrians looked concernedly at me but were too frightened of losing their own precarious grip to come to my aid. Eventually, and with great relief, I made it to the bottom of the hill, caught the train and changed at Lewes for Falmer.

Although, given the opportunity, I might have taken issue with Sir Basil Spence over the massiveness of the buildings he created for the university, I had always warmed to the red brick and to the exquisite landscaping of Stanmer Park, which I remembered from childhood. Now, in mid-December, both parkland and university looked lovelier than I remembered. The university especially, less that ten years old when I had first gone there, raw, imposing and looking as if it was still trying to impress, had now been established over twenty years, and it had mellowed. Each blade of grass, each flagstone, each pore of brick and mortar absorbed the fragile winter light and welcomed me home. And I never felt that more clearly than when I passed the circular Meeting House on my right, with its lozenges of coloured glass, where I'd married your dad five years before.

Because of somewhat bizarre train timetabling, I was very early and stopped at my old stamping ground, the School of Cultural and Community Studies. I had thought of simply biding my time, checking out old haunts deserted for the holidays, so I was thrilled to find that Hugh Young was there, in his room. He'd been my personal tutor, and one of my history tutors, and a very good one. He'd also been a good friend of Carl, the bloke I went out with most of the time I was at Sussex, who'd gone on to do a PhD at Cambridge.

The way to Hugh's door was virtually paved in lights, as he'd graduated to Dean of the Faculty status. I sat in his office and relaxed, while he told me what he'd heard about Carl, and I updated him on my teaching, my marriage, Benjamin and Sam, and your impending birth. He also said that he felt the course was a good one, that Karen was a really good tutor and that I'd get a lot out of it. The sun was still shining when I emerged to walk to the Education Development Building, feeling more than ever that I was coming home.

The interview itself was less of an interview than a chat. I had remembered Karen Thorpe, who was running the course, as a somewhat precious young woman in purple velvet jackets and flared trousers, with brassy hair hanging limply below her chin. Now, her hair had darkened and lost its metallic tone, and was softly cut in a bob. Her voice was relaxed rather than sounding forced out through her vocal chords. Her face was fuller. In the few encounters I had had with Karen in my last year at Sussex, I had admired her achievements, but that had been it. Now, I felt that we could be friends.

But what I actually remember most clearly about the interview is another of the women, who breastfed her ten-month-old baby daughter the whole time I was there. I immediately identified with her, and felt a rush of love for you, and the new life we were both on the verge of.

I came out certain that I would be offered a place on the course. There had been one sour note - lack of funding. The university had no money available, and the course cost over £400 a year - far more than I could afford. Karen suggested that I write to bodies that fund academic research, and wished me luck.

Suddenly, as I walked back through the campus, I noticed the weather change. Thick clouds covered the sky, and the wind became bitter. The grass too became greyish as if it resented being out in this sudden biting wind. The translucent windows of the Meeting House had now become lifeless eyes, set in sockets of gritty shells. It was as if all my former life, which less than an hour before had opened up and shown me a golden moment of divine possibilities, was now slamming a door in my face. I walked through the cheerless subway and sat on the station to wait for my train back to Hastings. A student walked over the iron bridge. The wind blew grey dust on my face. For the first time that day I thought about you properly - as yourself, rather than as an adjunct to my life. And I felt uneasy.

Back in Hastings, I had to go to the doctor's first to collect a note of introduction to the hospital. Mindful of the fact that I would probably have a wait in the hospital and that it would be uncomfortable because I'd need to have a full bladder, I decided to buy a book on the way. At that time, WH Smith was near the doctor's. I perused the shelves of general fiction, but nothing seemed to grab me. Then I wandered over to the detective novels, which was a strange thing to do, as it's not a genre I usually read. Eventually, realising there wasn't much time, I selected a PD James book - one of her Cordelia Grey novels, called "The Skull Beneath the Skin." In view of what was about to happen I could not have chosen anything more savagely or hideously appropriate. Either this was fate, or there are laws surrounding cause and effect of which we understand too little.

Standing waiting to pay for my purchase, I realised I needed the toilet and that it wouldn't wait until I got to the hospital, let alone allowed time for the scan. So after visiting the toilet at the doctor's when I collected my note, I bought a huge carton of Ribena, and drank it on the bus, hoping that it would go down quickly, but not too quickly.

It must have been another finger on the same hand of fate, or of coincidence, that had brought me to Dexter Hospital the previous day, and made sure this was not my first ever visit to a hospital that, up till only two weeks ago, I'd had no intention of ever entering as a patient. I went in through the main entrance, unaware that there was a side-entrance for ante-natal patients. It was through this that Tina entered after I'd been waiting about half an hour.

I thanked her for her concern in coming to see me now, and in ringing in the morning - and how grateful I had been on the glassy hill. I remember telling her how well the interview had gone, and a few other sundry exchanges were made before her children began demanding a lot of attention and she decided to take them home. I still think of Tina as the last of my friends to see me alive.

24 A Scan

All I needed was the love you gave
All I needed for another day
And all I ever knew
Only you

In the event, I nearly didn't have the scan. By quarter to four Tina had gone and I felt hot, bloated and extremely uncomfortable. The Ribena had certainly done the trick and I was crossing my legs one way and then the other. I was on the verge of getting up and leaving when the scanning sister came out - and took another patient in.

"Excuse me," I knew that my red face, caused by discomfort and indignation did me no favours, but I was determined to have my say - "my appointment was for three o'clock."

"Name?" This green-uniformed sister looked unsmiling through steel-framed glasses, her pale lips narrowing.

"Mrs. Sutherland."

"There's been some mistake, Mrs. Sutherland. Your appointment isn't until four o'clock." She merely gave me the information.

"But I have an appointment with Mr. Crosbie, the consultant, at four o'clock!" I said it too loudly, too triumphantly, flourishing my piece of paper like Neville Chamberlain.

"Mr. Crosbie," she informed me coolly, "isn't even in the building". By now, her mouth was little more than one straight line. I felt as if the air had been let out of me, and I sat down. The only part of me that seemed full was my bladder. The sister retreated into the scanning room. If I was not in in twenty-five minutes, I was going, I decided. Outside, the light, a granular grey when Tina had come to see me, had almost been drawn away.

Two minutes before my deadline, Sister Francis - I read her name badge this time - summoned me into the scanning room. Her anaemic lips looked a little fuller again, and some of the abrasive edge had gone from her manner, but it was still in a perfunctory way that she said -

"I can't promise you you'll have a perfect baby, like I could have at eighteen weeks."

"I understand that." I felt myself hardening. What did my decision to have my baby at home have to do with her?

Flat out on the bed, my oceanic stomach protrudes into the air. Sister Francis rubs cold jelly onto it, then I feel the scanner. Images begin to appear on the screen. I can see your spine very clearly.

"The baby is breech," she says, cursorily. Then she moves the scanner around more. All is silent. I can make out nothing clearly.

"Are you sure of your dates?"

"Yes."

All the unease which has lain at the back of my mind since the day I was told to rest because of the oedema, now hangs in the room. I simply wait for her to tell me something about my baby - something about you. Nothing happens.

Nothing happens except that she is putting the scanner into more and more unlikely positions - to try and find your head. Eventually she stops. Right up under my ribcage, on the right, I can see where your head is meant to be, but it won't come into focus. I can see my own ribs, and some kind of shadow. And that is it. There is nothing there. I know why. I do not want this knowledge. Every part of me that had known for months that I was carrying a damaged child came slap bang against the inevitable truth and knew there was no escape. Except in the waiting.

"Go and empty your bladder and I'll put you in the picture."

At the toilet, I pass masses of water yet relieve only my bladder. A weight hangs over me, but as yet, it has not fallen. Perhaps it will not fall. I can prolong this unknowing. I can prolong it. And if I can't, I am ready, because I know.

When I go back into the room, Sister Francis has a softer edge. She is still matter-of-fact, but not hostile. I sense that whatever she has to tell me, it will not be construed as my fault. I am matter-of-fact too. I can cope with anything. She says she thinks from the scan that there may be something wrong with the baby. I show no emotion. First, she says, she is sending me for an X-ray,

"Anencephaly." There is a whisper in my brain, but it is faint, bubbling beneath the surface, and I can make it stay there.

The X-ray, which involves lying face down, is extremely uncomfortable, but I remain very still. I know the dangers of X-rays for unborn babies. I know they would not be doing this without a very good reason.

"Anencephaly." The whisper is louder. It is threatening to break the surface.

I return to the waiting area. A few minutes later I see the radiologist go into the scanning room with my X-rays. She does not look at me on her way in or on her way out. I feel nothing. I know there is a pain associated with something I will not want to hear. I know there is hope, until the second I am told. I can almost hold out my hand to that hope. But I cannot make the effort. I am too lead heavy. Sister Francis pushes the metal handle and comes out through the wooden door. She knows she has to look at me, and she makes that effort. She attempts to steady me, by using my name - "Come in, Penelope" - but her mistaken use of this name, rather that Penny, which is how I am normally called, merely heightens the sense of unreality. Part of me looks on. This is happening to someone else who has a name like mine.

"Anencephaly." The word breaks the surface and is formed in my mind. The ripples that spread are infinite. The pain is unknown.

"I know," I tell myself. "But it's okay I'm calm. I needn't make a fool of myself in front of her."

"Penelope," she repeats when I am seated on the other side of her desk. "I'm sorry to have to tell you there's a gross abnormality here. It's incompatible with life. The baby is anencephalic. It means..."

"I know what it means. The baby has no skull, no proper brain." I realise that the Esther Rantzen programme is the only source I have of this knowledge. And suddenly, unexpectedly, the tears come. No amount of knowing anything could ever have prepared me for this. Wave after wave after wave - every moment of uneasiness, every hope, everything I had invested in the pregnancy and in you - all smashed into myriads of pieces to take in all in one go. It is hearing the word anencephaly that breaks me, hearing it from the irrefutable lips of Sister Francis. It had sounded so many times in my brain. But that was only the echo. This is the source. At the same time, I know that while my soul is bleeding, this is only an infinitely small first step. This is the rest of my life.

Sister Francis says nothing. She passes me her box of tissues. Between the first and second bouts of crying I remember our earlier antagonism. I feel I should apologise.

"I'm sorry. I knew what you were going to say when I was waiting out there. I was going to be so brave. I wasn't going to make a fool of myself like this."

"It's not the same as being told though," Sister Frances says sagely, gently, and for the first time I realise that to some extent she can empathise with what I'm going through. Another wave of anguish hits me, and I hear myself crying really loudly this time, and it's totally uncontrollable. There is no light left in the world outside. Only a little desk lamp sheds a pool of unreal light where I'm sitting. I hear words.

"Sometimes, Penelope, I hate this job. It's awful to have to give people news like this. And I had to give someone else similar news yesterday."

I cannot absorb this information. Someone else? No, this can never have happened to anyone else. Yes, intellectually I know that there are people who lose babies. I have met some. I have heard of others. But I cannot relate to the idea of any other human being experiencing such bitter, devastating and isolating grief. How can anyone be told something like this and go on living? Sometimes, even now, this returns as one of the unanswered questions of my life.

Though my eyes are like jellyfish, I take a quick look at Sister Francis. The lines around her mouth show relief, as though she would have found my bravery harder to handle - she can deal better with this flood of grief.

Then I say the first thing which shows, even then, how little I know of you, or of myself - how much, indeed, you have to teach me. Already, the initial grief of knowing you are lost to me is giving way to the sheer horror and terror of the monster, the freak, that I have bred. You have a deformed head - but you are not your deformed head. At that stage, I cannot understand this. All those disabled children that I had crossed the street to avoid were only a prelude to walking away from you - to wanting you, and your gross disfigurement, banished from me forever.

"I prefer it this way than to have to bring up a handicapped child."

"Yes, I'm sure."

Although this is true, I feel that I am doing Sister Francis a favour, in trying to look on something resembling a bright side. At least this way, I think, there is the cleanness and completeness of death. In the same way that once, there was a cleanness in having only two children, of a completed project. It seems strange that the end result should be the same, yet arrived at so devastatingly differently.

Had Sister Francis - or anyone - contradicted me at that stage, and told me that, once I had seen you and held you I would want you here, with me, in this world, on any terms, I would have thought it a joke sicker than the malformed child I carried inside me. I think of the Esther Rantzen programme again, and of the young mother who constantly gets her husband to draw pictures of their anencephalic baby because not knowing is worse than any reality would have been. It is beyond my comprehension. I feel sick to my womb.

Sister Francis, medical, practical, is beginning to address the issue of getting the baby out.

"I can arrange for you to see Mr. Crosbie soon. We'll keep you in and induce labour in the morning."

There is too much information. I address the only thought in my mind.

"I want a Caesarean." The tears have now stopped, but there are breaks between the words. My throat is choking. I cannot imagine any circumstances in which I would want a normal delivery for this gross abnormality. I am not having a baby, and to have this in the same way that Benjamin and Sam were born seems an obscenity. I cannot give birth to it, and don't expect this to be asked of me. All I want is to wake up and find it's been taken away.

"But it's incompatible with life," insisted Sister Francis, as though I hadn't understood. "You don't want to scar your uterus for a baby who will die." The relevance of this argument is totally lost on me. In the midst of all this, how could it possibly matter?

"I just want to wake up and find it's gone. I never want to see it, never want to know I had it. Just get over the operation."

I start crying again. Sister Francis seems to accept the reasonableness of what I am saying, but in fact it is a decision that neither of us can make, and she is prepared to leave it there. She has virtually done her bit.

"We'll see, then," she says. "You can talk it over with Mr. Crosbie."

The mention of Mr. Crosbie makes me remember that, had she taken two more minutes over the previous scan, I would now be at home, having walked back in ignorance through the murky, darkening streets. More than anything now, I want to be with your dad, to be with your normal, healthy brothers and prove to myself that that part of my life is more real than what is happening to me now.

"Can I go home?" I ask, more in hope than expectation.

"I don't think so, Penelope. With so much fluid, you could go into labour at any time. And because the baby's breech it could be dangerous." I suddenly realise that I have been going around for weeks carrying an unexploded time-bomb, and that I will never again see my home, or my children in it, until it has been made safe.

"Can I ring my husband and arrange things?"

"Of course." Her voice is almost inaudible. At the ends of her narrow lips there is a compassionate smile.

Silently, she passes me the phone. I speak to your dad slowly. I have to know that he has understood the first time, as I couldn't bear to repeat anything. I am also preparing myself to shoulder this grief alone, if I have to, knowing that it was me, and not him, that wanted the baby, and that now, I am leaving him to pick up the pieces. *This is not it, at all. This is not what I meant, at all.*

"So can you bring my night things round?"

"Of course. I'll be there as soon as I can."

"Oh - and could you bring me a recent photo of Benjamin and Sam? There's that one I had done recently in a studio. I feel the need to look at it."

"Okay" It is like your dad not to let bad news affect him until he can allow it to. He does that now, holding things together. Things have to be done - and it is impossible to know how he has taken the news.

Putting down the receiver, I feel that when I came to the hospital that afternoon I was holding several precious stones. By far the most precious was my daughter, but there was also the home delivery, the breastfeeding, the wholeness of myself and the name, Rebecca Louise. And, taken for granted, and therefore the smallest stone of all, was a healthy baby. Whereas the other stones were of jagged rose quartz, the last was a dull red, smooth pebble.

Now, one by one. I have had to throw them all away, but before I did, their relative value changed. The healthy baby stone has now changed to be the most achingly precious gift that there can be - a vibrantly red ruby. It has gone now, irretrievably mixed with all the pebbles on the lost beach of my life. But one searing question remains, and I have to ask,

"Could you tell from the scan whether the baby was a boy or a girl?"

"Probably a girl, my dear," replied Sister Francis gently. "They usually are."

This is not just the start of a personal unbearable grief; it is also a poke in the eye for everything I have come to believe about the wonder of women.

"I'll get someone to take you up to Louise ward," Sister Francis tells me, then looks baffled by the renewed sobs.

"Louise was going to be the baby's middle name," I explain.

"Oh, I'm so sorry, Penelope. We'll put you on another ward if you like."

"No, if you do that I'll always know that I deliberately avoided it. I'll be okay"

Sister Francis writes up some more notes then disappears to find a duty sister, who takes me to another room. Sister Francis says goodbye, and wishes me well. The duty sister, with large blue eyes, dimples and smooth skin on a round face, has one of the kindest faces I have ever seen, yet a fine line is set through the centre of her mouth.

I repeat my plea for a Caesarean, while she takes my details, but like Sister Francis, she firmly insists that it is not a good idea.

"You do realise this baby is going to die, don't you?" she asks the question as softly as she can but with firmness, so that, had I been under any illusions about the outcome, they could never have emanated from her.

"Yes, and that's why I want the Caesarean."

"And that's why it's not worth scarring your uterus for the future, you know." Suddenly I am aware of the implications of what she is saying, and the futility of her words. How could the future of my poor uterus possibly matter? It is carrying something hideous, deformed - I blame it as much as I despise you, for containing something so gross, and soon to be dead. It is totally inconceivable that anything good and healthy could ever come out of it again. After this, there could be no more life, either for me or through me.

In my next memory, I am lying on my bed in Louise ward. I have my own room, and for this, I am extremely grateful, and find out later that it is hospital policy to put those of us who lose our babies into this ward. I also discover later from Alison, who used to be a nurse in the local area, that this is also a private room. I would never have associated this with the glossy BUPA images: it seems to be aeons since the high-ceilinged, square Victorian room was painted shell pink. Paint is peeling from the walls and the lino is shabby. Yet it is the kind of room I need. It's what I think I deserve.

Your dad hasn't arrived yet, and I am still wearing the blue pinafore dress lent to me by Sharon Clayton, one of the mums at St. Andrews toddler group.

I have worn it a lot - nearly as much as I wore Rosie's smock - because I really liked it. It's made of a kind of denim fabric, with red and yellow embroidery on the yoke and straps. Now, I recall that I was also wearing it when Dr Walker first discussed the excess fluid and oedema, before I went to Springles restaurant that dreadful afternoon. Immediately superstitious, I now regard it as an unlucky dress, and want to rip it off, as if that would change what has happened, where I am, or how I got here.

Someone knocks and kindly leaves me sandwiches that remain uneaten. Then your dad arrives, with Benjamin and Sam. I reach out and hold them, needing the life they provide, and their proximity to the life force, but inside, part of me holds back. I am frightened of contaminating them with the death and deformity I am carrying. They are too young for tears, to understand the scope of the loss. They have already accepted, in a matter-of-fact way, that the baby has not grown properly in mummy's tummy and that she will be coming home without it. Your dad asks after my comfort. He has brought me everything I need - for the hospital stay. I cannot tell how he feels, and I do not want to know, in case he tells me all I've done is ruined everybody's lives. After they have gone I remove the hated pinafore and put on my nightdress. I fastidiously arrange a few objects he has brought on the bedside table, including the photo of your brothers. They are so open, so honest, so beautiful and so perfect that, although I need to know the photo is there, I cannot bear to look at it. I walk along the corridor to the bathroom. Locked inside, alone, I see a long mirror, and, once I have seen it, I cannot ignore the full-length view of my body. The bump, which is you, looks enormous. I had carried it once so proudly, as I had all my pregnancies. Now its futility mocks all I ever wanted in having another baby. This is not a baby at all. And then, perhaps for the first time since I found out about your condition, I feel you kick. I do not want this reminder. Of this kicking, of this movement, I want only one thing - that it should cease.

"Why can't you just die?" I address you, alone with me in that spartan bathroom with its strip lighting. "Why can't you just die?" The tears come again - this time angry, frustrated. They are all for me. There can be none for you. You, as far as I am concerned, are not even human. And you have done this to me.

There is another mirror on the opposite wall: in this one, I can see just my face. I look at myself for a long time, as if studying my own face will give my some clue, will show me some truth about myself previously hidden, or will somehow explain all this to me. Somehow, I expect to look different from how I looked this morning - when I set off, what seems like a lifetime ago, for my interview.

My pretty, but somewhat bland features, look steadily back at me. I do not look my age - I never have. Pregnancy, and especially the oedema, has filled out my face, and if anything that has made me look more childlike. I have big blue-grey eyes, inherited from my father, a small nose and pretty normal lips. My light brown hair is long at the moment, and curly at the ends - the remains of that perm I had shortly before you were conceived. My cheeks are reddish, very much like Tina's, and I will clearly never attain my adolescent aim of looking pale and interesting. But in my way, I realise I look as normal and average, after all, as Helen Jones, or Alison. And that is it. I am going through an incomprehensible hell and apparently I have nothing to show for it. Listlessly, I return to my room. The frustration has ebbed away. All I feel now is a sense of submitting to something far bigger than I am - just in the way that allowed me to become pregnant with you in the first place. In letting go, emotions, for the moment, leave me. It seems there is nothing to do. I look through my belongings. I have one book - "The Skull beneath the Skin"- which I cannot begin to face reading. I lie on my back and, motionless, stare at the ceiling.

I don't know how long I have been there before a nurse comes to find me and suggests I might have a television. I don't even have the will to tell her I don't want this intrusion and entertainment, and to let her get it seems the way of least resistance. She returns shortly with a black-and-white portable which she plugs in. The Russell Harty Show is on. It is at once a lacerating dislocation to be reminded that out there is another world untouched by hideous events, and at the same time, comforting to know that life goes on in its routines. The nurse leaves the room. Russell Harty introduces his guests, The Flying Pickets. They sing a song - "Only You" - which seems to have been written specially for me, and whose haunting qualities will be associated with you for as long as I live.

Some time later another nurse and doctor arrive. I still haven't seen Mr. Crosbie. Although I'm special, it would seem, there should not be any gynaecological complications associated with the delivery. The doctor says I will need a pessary to open the cervix, and they will decide later whether to put it in tonight or in the morning. He also suggests an epidural- an option which I so far hadn't considered. That way, he says, I will be spared both the pain of a difficult labour, and the long-term problems of a Caesarean. And I do not have to see the baby if I do not want to.

This seems the best compromise. I feel part of me sinking again as I agree to yield yet another of my rose quartz stones - that of a natural birth. Now, it seems, all that is left of what I wanted is only in my head, and that's where it has to stay. Reality is only a bizarre mockery.

At about nine o'clock, your dad comes back, having got our next-door neighbour to babysit for an hour or so. I cry onto his shoulder. Although he has not abandoned himself to any grief, I have the feeling that this is because he has to keep me and the boys together, and be practical. Instinctively I know that it's not because he doesn't care, or that he blames me. He has made arrangements for Benjamin and Sam for the following day. He has got time off work and he will be at the birth. I say that if the baby is a girl, we might call her Louise. I don't want to use up the Rebecca - not for this baby, and somehow, the name has chosen itself. He, too, thinks it's a lovely name. And although I do not consciously acknowledge it, there is a thought fluttering on the edges of consciousness that somehow the name Rebecca might still have some kind of future.

After your dad has gone, I doze off. I think, as the medical staff clearly do, that if only I'd had a scan at eighteen weeks, all this would have been avoided. You would have been out of the way by now, I would never have had to confront this, and I could have got on with the rest of my life. I could even have been pregnant again by now.

At ten o'clock I am roused from my doze by the drinks coming round, and the duty doctor returning to examine me and tell me that I won't need a pessary until the morning. I put out the light and doze a bit more. I don't dare abandon myself to sleep. I can't bear the thought of losing consciousness to wake up and discover, all over again, the horror of what is happening to me.

Part Four

Birth and Afterbirth

25 The Day of Delivery

Looking from a window above
It's like a story of love
Can you hear me?

Despite myself, I do fall asleep, but when I come round in the morning, I do not have to re-remember the nightmare of yesterday. Somehow I remained conscious of it all the time I was asleep. It is Wednesday, 14th December, 1983. Having been woken at six, I have been pretty much left alone for two hours. At about eight o'clock I am given another examination by another doctor I have never seen before, and my pessaries are inserted. Then your dad arrives, and we go downstairs into something optimistically called the First Stage room.

Some time later, the scent of an exclusive aftershave filters into this austere room, heralding the arrival of Mr. Crosbie, so anxiously anticipated the previous day. He is quite a short, tanned man, with a soft West Country burr at the edges of his voice. His entire body seems to exude affluence and comfort.

He is abrupt, but not unkindly so. He is merely being professional. He has to be there because this is abnormal, but I should not present with the kinds of interesting difficulties that actually justify his enormous salary. He can also afford to be abrupt, I realise, because he knows exactly what he is doing. He skims my notes for only a few seconds, but I can tell from the way he puts his hands on me that he has not only absorbed all the information, but can act on it. His hands move skilfully over my abdomen. Immediately, he can feel which way the baby is lying. He also informs the attendant nurse, as he carries out the second internal of the morning, that I should have been given the pessaries the night before, and I am glad I am not the doctor who decided it could wait. I am also glad that the doctor got it wrong, because they have already started to burn, and I would not have wanted to put up with that all night. However, he still concludes that in the light of my obstetric history, I should not be in labour for too long. This is the first comment he has addressed to me. He has looked inside me first.

He orders the nurse to fit me up with a portable drip, and at this stage, I ask about the epidural that had been suggested the previous evening. Actually getting the labour started is acting as an anaesthetic for the emotional pain. but suddenly I am frightened of the labour itself - of going through the deepest physical pain anyone can experience, without the exhilaration of a new life to come. And as I explain to Mr. Crosbie -

"I'm okay when they're my contractions - when I know it's my body doing it. But when the syntocinon gets to work, I have no control over the pain."

"Yes, that will be fine," his chocolate-smooth voice replies. He turns to the nurse. "You can contact the anaesthetist."

"Fine, Mr. Crosbie." I half-expect her to curtsy.

"I will come in later, to see how things are going," he informs me. He departs. The smell of his after-shave lingers in the room. He has kept his expensive camel-coloured cashmere coat on all the time he has been in there. I like the air of professional detachment exuded by him, and conveyed to his staff. It is exactly congruent with how I am feeling as I watch my arm being invaded, so the only thing I can be attached to is the drip. My emotions and my body belong to someone else. At the same time, there is some excitement in the room, some anticipation that something is happening. It is almost like giving birth.

Despite Mr. Crosbie's predictions, and the drip, things actually take a long time to get underway - probably because I was not given the pessaries the night before. That too, though, is characteristic of my labours. The previous two started with a torrent of water and then nothing for several hours. I soon feel the restrictions of the first stage room, which contains three beds and so, although the drip is portable, I cannot move around freely, which I suppose defeats the whole object of putting me on a portable drip in the first place.

Your dad and I talk in a desultory way for the next hour or so, then I am taken into the labour room, where you will actually be born. I know that I am nowhere near giving birth, so I wonder if the hospital staff have some idea that this move may psychologically help me hurry up a bit. I am getting the impression that although they are sympathetic, they think that, the sooner this is all over, the better it will be for everyone. I am inclined to agree.

At about half past eleven, another doctor presents himself. He too is short, but very pale, with yellow hair. His bottom lip seems to be unnecessarily slack. Much of his face is pitted and two livid spots are developing just above his collar. I have long since given up trying to read the names of the people who are caring for me. Including Mr. Crosbie, this is the fourth doctor who has given me an internal since I arrived at the hospital- the third that morning. His brief is to find out if I am ready to have my waters broken. He too is abrupt, but not with professional integrity. This borders on rudeness. Again, with a nurse at the other side of the bed, he feels inside me without having once looked at my face. And whereas Mr. Crosbie's hands had moved quickly but competently, this man's feel as though he thinks he is handling steak.

From the moment he begins, I know I am not ready for the waters to be broken. If I were, it would not hurt so much. Then he reaches in with an instrument that reminds me of a crochet hook. Previously silent while all this poking was going on, I cry out.

"Be quiet please. I cannot do the examination if you call out."

"Use the entonox," says the nurse, slapping the mask over my face. I take great drafts of the stuff.

Suddenly, and probably for the last time, I feel you kick. I have taken so much, and I cannot take any more. I feel very woozy, and take the mask off. I cannot take this unnecessary pain - going through all this for a baby that will die. There is no other way of expressing what I feel, other than tears. I sob effusively onto your dad's shoulder.

Incredulous, the doctor looks up from his work, across at the nurse on the other side of the bed.

"Why is she crying?"

The nurse takes a deep sigh.

"I think she's in shock."

"Oh."

He cannot, or does not want to, handle anything resembling emotion. Still addressing my vagina rather than me, he amplifies his request.

"Do you think you could stop crying while I finish my examination?" I am normally so docile and meek around anyone in the medical profession, but through the walls of pain I sob,

"No, no I can't. Not yet."

With an indignant sigh, he removes his hand and the crochet hook and sweeps out of the room. He has failed. My pain has made him fail. Later that day I hear he has been bitten by a dog and needed treatment in casualty.

Another couple of hours go by. Your dad goes for some lunch. I am in yet another pink emulsioned room. They seem to be a feature of historic moments in this pregnancy. The only windows in the high-ceilinged, square room - this hospital seems to specialise in these too - are right at the top. I can see a few pewter-grey clouds. There is no sun.

Always, my eyes cannot help coming back to the pictures which decorate the walls. They are pictures of healthy babies - obviously put up to encourage women in labour - a reminder to push harder, as that's what they would soon have. There are babies of different ages, from newborn through to smiling and mobile babies. Healthy babies. Alive babies. The sort of baby I am not going to have. And they are the only animated aspect of the room. They are only magazine photos, and I don't know why no-one thought to take them down, knowing it was me in there for the day.

Your dad returns, closely followed by Mr. Crosbie, who does another external version, confirming the position of the baby. Now, it's his turn with the crochet hook. This time I am ready, and feel only a release of built-up pressure as gallons of amniotic fluid shoot out over the bed and onto the floor. Mr. Crosbie leaps out of the way. The fluid misses his camel coat but splashes on his soft black leather shoes. "There," he says, looking at me, "that should feel easier now." From the softness of his voice, I imagine that the nurse has briefed him on my last obstetric encounter.

"Thank you " I return his gaze with gratitude.

Any lingering hope I might have had the night before that somehow it had all been a mistake; that the baby would come out and we would find that, after all, it was all right, has been completely laid to rest by actually seeing all that liquor. I remember from before what it should look like - colourless and clear. This is yellowish, like something fetid, indicating that something is very wrong.

The nurse comes back in with a mop. Like many nurses, she has a slim, clipped-in waist. Lots of dark, shiny, ebullient curls frame her cap. While she clears up the mess, she tells me that they are going to turn up the syntocinon on the drip, to speed up the labour, and that the anaesthetist is on his way.

Almost as soon as she has finished saying this, he turns up. For someone whose title seem to be pronounced in virtually hallowed tones, he turns out to be a somewhat silly, jokey man, who boasts about not having done one of these for at least six months, and isn't sure if he can remember what to do.

I feel the prick of a needle near the base of my spine, and it is not long before my legs go numb. I hadn't been prepared for my legs to look so normal and to feel so weird - so elephantine - as though they are somewhere up on the ceiling. It also occurs to me that I will no longer be able to feel you kicking, and I am glad about that. The nurse turns up the syntocinon. I can cope with this because I have no feeling - of any sort.

I lay unmoving on the bed. A circular wall clock, with a grey face and black hands, moves round, but time means nothing here. Tina has had your brothers for the day, and your dad will soon have to go and collect them, give them their tea and put them to bed. After that, Maxine and Jeff, a couple he knows from work, whom I've met a few times and like, are coming to babysit. Even though I can feel nothing, I know he can safely be away for a few hours, before anything happens.

Already, it is only the street lights that penetrate the thick winter darkness outside. This really is the death of the year. Your dad puts on the coat which he wore throughout the first winter I knew him, nearly six years ago. He was proud of the fact that he had bought it at Horne's, albeit in a sale. From the outside it still looks fine - comfortable to wear, and it's only the two of us who know how shabby the lining is. It's one of the jobs I have been meaning to sort out, and have never got round to. There is something I need to say before he goes. In the midst of all this, there is something I want to get sorted.

He bends down to kiss me. Our lips brush gently, with an untold acknowledgement of all that is happening. His moustache tickles slightly. I have never quite got used to the contrast between its silkiness and bristly, cropped edges. Then as he straightens up, I say, looking past him to the pictures on the wall,

"One day, when this is over, I would like to have another baby." I am prepared to give him time to think about this. After all, I feel, in a sense, he has got what he wanted - there is going to be no third baby. The concept of Benjamin and Sam remains intact. And I don't really know why I've said it, because objectively, I cannot relate to any future. In some obscure way, I am reaching out for a sense of healing. But he replies almost immediately,

"Yes, I can relate to that." And for the first time in a long time, I remember what hope means, and it is not just for me, but for my continued relationship with him.

He leaves. It is about five o'clock. There are two new nursing staff -one nurse and one sister - outside the delivery room, and I get the feeling they will be there now for the duration. It is with a shock that I realise that most of the women who have taken care of me since last night are, actually, as these, midwives. One of them moves me on to my side, because I cannot move myself. It is my left side, from which I can see the clock. For the next hour, I watch the minutes go round, and round, and round. Fascinated by childbirth, I have read many descriptions of labour - in fiction and real accounts, written by women, written by men. At the extremes, it is sheer hell or a totally awesome psychosexual experience. It can, in a perverse way, be both. But this is simply nothing. As the clock goes round, all that seems to happen is that the two midwives - and it takes two of them - periodically move me into a sitting position and place a bedpan under my bottom. I have no feeling, to know whether I have used it or not. I am temporarily (I hope) disabled by my deformed baby. For her, the disability is permanent, and a death sentence.

One of the midwives, the archetypal Girl with Green Eyes, examines me at about twenty past six. She addresses me in a soft Irish voice.

"We're getting on quite well now, you know. There's definite progress." I decide that she's still pretty young to have acquired this medically patronising use of the word "we" but then realise that to her it does apply - she does feel that all of us in these rooms are in this together.

"How far open is the cervix?"

"About two centimetres." She's right. That's some progress. Not a lot. Carry on going at this rate and I'll still be in here tomorrow tea time. But as I do know from experience, the speed of the early phases of labour does not always bear much relation to that of later ones.

"The trouble is," she says, "that the baby can't do anything for itself. And of course, there's no head to push out, so it will take a long time."

"And I won't even know when I go into transition, or when I want to push."

"No, you won't. I'm sorry," she added, genuinely. "I'll come back and examine you at half past eight."

She returns my whale-like body to the left side again. I have two hours to wait, and that's just for the next examination. Two hours before we can see how long it will be before I can get rid of the freak inside me, and have it taken away. It is the first time since labour began that I have really articulated this thought in my head.

Although I can't feel anything, after about an hour, I am aware that I need a change of position. Feeling like something being grilled, I ask to be turned. This time it's the sister who comes to attend to me. She looks about my age. Her hair was coloured some time before and there are still some brassy traces of dye. Like me, she has short fingers. She turns me over, then as she does so, takes the opportunity to have a quick look to see what is happening. She reports that she can see "two little feet" dangling down.

And what the dead had no speech for, when living,
They can tell you, being dead: the communication
Of the dead is tongued with fire beyond the language of the living.

If there was a single moment that changed forever the meaning of your life for me, that was it. The previous day, you had changed from being all that would fulfil every dream I ever had, to being a gross abnormality that made me feel sick to my soul. Now, the midwife had seen "two little feet." For the last twenty-four hours, I had been unable to think of any part of you as being in any way "normal" - you were too abhorrent to be thought of in any other terms than as a grossly deformed head. Now, I had to accept the fact that you were actually a baby. A poorly baby, yes, but none the less a baby. At last. My baby.

I am about to deliver. Everything suddenly happens. Someone goes away to ring your dad, muttering something about how they hope he gets here in time. I am moved into a delivery position. The midwife does another internal examination and discovers an anterior lip. Had I been able to feel anything, I would have had to pant like mad, and wait for it to sort itself out before I could give myself over to pushing. As it is, I cannot feel the urge to push so even this quite frequent complication of labour is irrelevant.

Your dad arrives and quickly puts on the hospital gown that he must, apparently, wear for the delivery. He looks, literally, like a delivery boy, but of bread rather than babies. And then I look into his face.

"What on earth is wrong with your eyelashes and eyebrows? Have you singed them or something?" Some of the lashes on his left eye seem considerably curtailed. His eyebrows - curiously dark, like Sam's, for one so fair - are the same, although some of the hairs curl round implausibly. He reluctantly tells me,

"I leaned over the fireguard to light the gas fire and the flames leapt out into my face."

I know I should be worried. I know he could have been badly hurt - as he reminds me now, in a somewhat bruised tone. And all I can do, thinking about the whoosh of the fire, and how ridiculous he looks with his hospital gown and stubbly eyebrows, is giggle. I am about to deliver a deformed baby and this is all I can think about.

Unfortunately, it's the dog doctor who comes back in to supervise the delivery, his right hand appropriately bandaged. Because of the darkness of the room though, in which the only lighted area is my birth canal, he seems to recede into the background. The sister tells him about the anterior lip, but he maintains that, because of the condition of the baby's head, I am ready. I no longer feel the remotest impulse to laugh. He turns to both nurses and asks if they would like to deliver the baby. They say that they would.

"Now," Again, he addresses the pool of light rather than me, "you can push when you feel a contraction." I look into the dark space from which his thin voice seems to come, in amazement. Can he possibly have forgotten?

"I can't feel anything, because of the epidural." And it is with irritation on his face that he steps out of the shadow to put his hand on my abdomen and inform me, "You're having a contraction now."

I start to push into my vagina. Although I can't feel anything, I try to imagine where the muscles are, as Jayne has taught me. And the result is staggering. In one push, the baby's legs and bottom are born. The dog doctor moves away, and lets the sister take over. "We're nearly there," she tells me. And even in the moments you are being born, I have to know.

"What is it?"

"A girl."

Somewhere deep in my being, I scream in silence. I know that, at some stage, I will have to give voice to that scream. But other things are going on, and I know this is not the time. As you come out, I want to see you delivered.

I look down, between my legs. Your legs are tucked under you. I can see your bottom. Then the other nurse, monitoring my abdomen, alerts me to another contraction. With that push, I see your little back come out. You will be born with your face turned towards the bed. And I don't know what is happening now. Is this an inordinately long contraction, or should I stop pushing and await another one? Or is another one already starting?

"Go on," your dad says, and there is a look of total wonder and amazement on his face. This is a birth of one of his children - as much as any of the others.

"It's wonderful," he whispers, reverently.

"Go on," the nurse softly echoes, and I push for the last time. And this bit, I cannot face. Before your head comes out, I turn my own away. But your dad doesn't stop looking. He actually sees the whole of you born.

As soon as you are delivered, they deftly scoop you up and take you away to where we cannot see you. I know you are dead. I remember how blue you were, lying between my legs, still not separate from me, but not moving. Never to move again. But in the few moments I have seen you so far, there has been no horror, only a profound sense of perfect peace. For the first time in my life I have understood the peace that passes understanding. And it is you who have shown it to me.

After a few silent minutes, the sister returns.

"Do you want to see the baby?"

I hesitate. I still don't want to have anything to do with your deformed head, but I do want to be with you. I am having difficulty reconciling these two concepts. At the same time, I am on an immediate post-natal high - the same euphoria, the same elation, that accompanies any birth. It is the last thing I expected to feel.

"She's got a lovely little face. We can cover her head."

"Yes, all right then." At least, this way, I can be with you. I do not have to see what I do not want to. Your dad nods in agreement.

And so, my love, you are brought to me. And, like any mother anywhere, I hold out my arms for my new infant and you are solemnly put into them. I look down at your face, and although there is nothing to be seen above the eyebrows, it is the most perfect and beautiful little face imaginable. It conveys, even through eyes that have never opened, only dignity, innocence and that profound sense of peace.

I am moved beyond emotion. The unutterable mysteries of birth and death are here, inextricably joined, enfolded in my arms. You are in a different world - only just, I can sense that - and I feel that it is you who regret that you cannot take me into your world, rather than me, that I cannot bring you into mine. Your face is full of ancient wisdom accepting that, simply, this was how it had to be, and that you have that most priceless of gifts, which I may somehow approach but will never fully comprehend - an understanding of why.

As I take the time to absorb the immanence of all this, I become more aware of the details of you - all the things that make you our daughter, rather than any other baby, living or dead. It still comes as something of a surprise when I look at your face and discover that you look just the same as your brothers when they were born, with the same chubby face and receding chin. I hadn't 14.   expected you to look so much like one of our children, and now, I'm so glad that you do, that you are already so much a part of our family. Then I notice there is a strand of hair poking out from the little white hood they have managed to find to cover your poor head - and, where your brothers' hair was Lesley white, this is very dark. So you got your hair from my mother- almost black, sultry, straight hair, inclined to go prematurely grey.

So this is who you are. It is not with the euphoria I once imagined in these unique moments that I discover this, but in a deep silence that echoes inside me, in the place from where you have come. I know you, as surely as if I were to bring you up myself.

Then, with reverence, and keeping your little hood in place, I undo the covers they have put round you. I know this time with you will never come again, and I must learn as much as I can in the time that is left to us. Tasting every moment, I look at your little body and run my hands over it. Although I am beyond feeling, I still realise how achingly like a normal baby you actually are. Vernix covers your skin, and I bow my head. The smell of newborn babies.

You are the tiniest baby I have seen, weighing less than five pounds, which is why Sister Francis asked me yesterday if I was sure about my dates. Yet you too seem to have the same oedema that has given so many problems: I suppose that, if you were unable to digest the fluid, it built up in you too. Your dad remarks on your chunky arms and legs, and I smile up at him, and then at you. Your legs too are the same shape as your brothers', with the knock knees inherited from me, given in turn by my mother. Then, before putting the covers back, I check your genital area just once more. My daughter. I hold you out to your dad. He takes you with the same gentleness and reverence.

The sister puts her head round the door. She has not wanted to intrude. In fact, I don't remember at what stage all the medical staff left - it just seemed so natural to be given this private time with you. She asks if we would like to have a photo taken. Yes please. I now want to preserve all the memories I can. Thisremains the only photo of you in existence. Actually, it took some trouble to get. Your dad gave you back to me, and we composed ourselves to look solemnly at the baby in a way we considered becoming for posterity. (If this sounds in any way flippant, I say it only because our beings had been taken to somewhere utterly new, and we had no known body language to express how we really felt .)

So I hold you for a long time in that posed solemn way while the sister tries for three photos - and nothing happens. There is a flash of light, then nothing. No picture.

"Hang on a minute" she says, and comes back a couple of minutes later with another camera. She finds us ostensibly in the same position. The only difference is that your mouth has now come open and I have found it impossible to shut it. Once again, tragedy is teetering on the edge of farce. I'm not sure how much longer I can hold out.

"I know this one works," she proclaims, and triumphantly takes the photo.

"Shall we have another one?" And she tries to take one just of Mother and Daughter. But we should have known better than to try our luck. At that stage the second camera packs up too. For some reason, you are fated to have only one precious photo of your existence.

Although I am pleased we have the photo, somehow taking it has broken the spell of those early moments with you. It's not the ridiculous circumstances of the photo - you with your mouth open, your dad with his singed eyebrows, me without any feeling in my legs, posing for minutes and minutes, - it is simply that with the click of the camera, I know that I have learnt everything in that early encounter with you that you could teach me. I know that the staff will allow me to keep you with me as long as I want, but it now seems pointless. I can never feed you, change you, wash you - all those relentless aspects of caring for a baby, after the first euphoria has worn off, are to be denied me. There is a lot still to be revealed to me from this encounter, but it will be unfolded through the rest of my life. You have to go on into your world, and I have to soldier on as best as I can in mine. I turn to your dad.

"I think I'm ready to let her go now."

"Yes," he agrees. He goes into the other room. The Girl with Green Eyes follows him back, and there is sadness in the tread of her flat black shoes around the bed. "Are you sure?" she asks softly. "Yes" we both say together. We both brush your cheek and say goodbye.

I still have not seen your head. Now it is too late, and I don't know whether I will regret this or not. I give you to her, and she looks at you as if you are a child of her own.

Then, the two midwives return and go about the business of finishing off this labour. The placenta is delivered - "it's perfectly normal," says the sister, and I am dismantled from the artificiality of the syntocinon and epidural drips. I don't know how long it will be before I will be able to feel my legs again.

After that, as with any normal delivery, I am given a cup of tea, which at the time, I really enjoy. But soon after, I am very sick - so suddenly, that there is no time to call out. The Girl with Green Eyes arrives to clear up the second copious amount of fluid that I have deposited on the floor that day. I am less upset by the mess than why they think I made it. I go to great lengths to reassure them that it had nothing to do with seeing the baby.

"I know that," she reassures me. Her voice has the softness of spring water. "It's a common reaction after an epidural."

I suppose they don't tell you this - or make contingency plans - in case you then make it happen. At least, presumably, the epidural drug is receding from my body. She looks up at me as she completes cleaning up the mess.

"We have done a card for Louise. Would you like it?"

"Yes please," your dad and I say together. She returns with a pink card. All your birth details are recorded. They have obviously filled most of it out before, and then added your name when it was known to them, as it is written in different handwriting, and with a different pen. I can see now, as I could then, that this could be construed as a cruel travesty of a normal birth, but I have never seen it that way. It is simply a record of the details of my baby. About the last thing of any significance that happens in the room is that an ancillary worker comes in to give me a wash. She wears a dark green uniform. She has grey hair and a very short neck, which seems rooted in her shoulders.

She too has an Irish accent. She reminds me of one of the cleaning women I knew years before, when I lived in hall of residence, who was called Mrs. Malone, and was consequently known as Molly.

"It's very quiet out there tonight," she tells me, nodding in the direction of the adjoining room. "It always is, when something like this happens." So already it is happening. We cannot say 'when a baby dies.' We have to say, 'something like this.' While she uses the one pool of light in the room to work by, I want to go out there and tell them "It's all right. It's okay Really it is. You can celebrate like you normally do."

I don't, because I don't want them to think me insensitive. What I don't know is that the delivery itself is merely a figure in a curtain swaddling itself round emotions that, as yet, I cannot afford myself to feel. I do not have the remotest idea that this is what's happening, except that I vaguely recall feeling (or rather not feeling) something like this when my dad - your grandad - died. Relatives wept around the grave while I looked on, wondering why they were crying. I wasn't being brave - or at least, not through choice. As the curtain started to tear, sometime later, I realised that, what I had done by instinct was protect myself. I cannot see this now - and that is for the best. In the meantime, all I want to do is reassure everyone.

Clean and comfortable, and wearing a crisp new hospital gown, I am ready to be moved back to Louise ward, and to say goodbye to the sister, The Girl with Green Eyes and Molly. They have steered me through some of the most momentous hours of my life, and I don't even know their names.

27 Jenny

We die with the dying:
See, they depart, and we go with them.
We are born with the dead:
See, they return, and bring us with them.

I am taken back up to Louise ward on the trolley, but the movement makes me feel sick. This time though, there is some warning, and I throw up into a stainless steel bowl before being put back into bed. The feeling is beginning to return to my legs, and they tingle a bit, not unpleasantly. I remark on this to the nurse who is sorting me out.

"Thank goodness for that. I thought I might be paralysed for life." I smile, glad to have made a joke of my fear. She laughs a bit, shrugging off any suggestion of the kind. She asks me if I am comfortable. I settle down in the bed. Your dad gives me a tender goodbye kiss and returns home, through the bitter night, to be with our living children.

Tonight, I know, I will be able to let myself sleep. When I wake up, and consciousness returns, I will be able to deal with what has happened. This is something I could never imagine, before you came to me. And as I drift off to sleep, it occurs to me that perhaps the medical profession are wrong, and perhaps this, in some way, is for the best.

I have, at least, had a baby. A dead baby, but a baby, nonetheless. A poor thing, but mine own. A baby I have held close to me. A baby I have named. A baby whose body I have explored. A baby who has taught me more in a few hours than I have probably learnt in most of my lifetime. And if I had had the routine scan at eighteen weeks, it would have picked up your "gross abnormality," and the pregnancy would have been terminated, because your condition was "incompatible with life." You would have remained a monster forever. I would have been afraid of you forever, and you would have remained only your condition - nothing more. Only this way can there be healing. This way, you are an accepted part of me and of all my family. I fall asleep quite easily. The next thing I know it is the middle of the night and I am suddenly wide awake. I switch on the bedside light, and look at my watch. Quarter to three. Becoming aware of my body - and my legs are fine now, to my relief - I discover it has several needs and that sleep will not return until they are met. I am amazed to discover that I am desperately hungry. I also need a bedpan, and my mouth feels foul. I want to clean my teeth.

When I ring the bell, it is two nurses who come to my aid. I ask for the bedpan first, because this seems, to me, the most understandable of my requests. While I am using it, I ask if I could possibly clean my teeth, and then add:

"I know this probably sounds really callous. Perhaps I shouldn't want to eat now. But I'm starving."

They are very understanding, and say it so happens that tonight, I'm lucky. There is some salad left in the fridge. One of them deals with the cleaning up process, while the other sorts out the food. Then, my mouth fresh and clean, they leave me to dine in peace. That meal, eaten alone, in an austere hospital room on a midwinter's night, lives still in my memory. Tomatoes have never tasted or smelled so redly, roundly, sweet, the bloom of coldness still on their skins. I also wolf down the ham (I wasn't vegetarian then) and some bread and butter. I lay my knife and fork neatly on the empty white plate, place it on my bedside table, put the light out again and sleep well for the second time that night.

As I start to come round the following morning, I think I can hear crying coming from the room next to me. I have seen no other patients since coming to Louise ward. But as I become more fully awake it stops, and I am not sure if I have heard it or not. It reminds me of the crying of Colin in The Secret Garden.

After breakfast - and I face this as heartily as the proverbial condemned man - your dad comes back, with fresh clothes. He has sensibly brought skirts with elasticated waists, which I can get into now, but couldn't wear towards the end of the pregnancy. This morning, he has left your brothers with Alison, and already I feel blessed to have so many friends who are willing to help. He has also had a word with Alison's vicar husband, Michael. who has offered to lead a blessing service that afternoon in the hospital chapel, if we would like. I agree immediately. It is a long while since I have had any contact with organised religion, but you are certainly part of something spiritual, beyond my understanding, and this is a way of acknowledging that. Because of my upbringing, it's what I have access to. Feeling, in my semi-familiar clothes as if I am making a new beginning, I go with your dad to the administrator's office to collect your birth/death certificate.

We wait in a corridor, and the registrar appears at a little window. Despite the fact that I do most of the talking, for patriarchal reasons, your dad has to be put on the certificate as the informant, and his paternity rights recognised. Because you were still-born, you are not allowed to be named. I think this is grossly unfair, and say so, but the registrar looks at me as if, because I am in the throes of grief, I am somehow demented and unable to think clearly. She reminds me that it's not long since still-born babies were given no certificate at all, which implies I should be grateful, and gratuitously reminds me "after all, the baby is dead, my dear" suggesting that it might be better if all this went unacknowledged and was swept under the carpet, as it always used to be. When I was someone else -i.e. up to yesterday evening - I would have agreed with her.

She also looks astonished when I say that I don't want the hospital to "deal with the body." I don't enquire too closely what this means - in fact, I don't enquire at all - but it certainly doesn't sound too pleasant. Guided partly by what I remember from watching "The Lost Babies," but increasingly by a developing awareness of what I really want, and what I know is best for all of us, I make a clear statement.

"I - we - want the baby to be buried." I have had to summon up something resembling courage to get this far, and I don't want a battle, but I have to defend all our rights. The registrar continues to look at me with a mixture of pity and wariness, but she has used up her trump card of reminding me that the baby is dead.

"I want there to be a piece of land - even if it's a small one - that is the baby's, and that will be there forever. Whenever I think of her, there will always be a place that she will be, as well as in our hearts."

"Fine," she says softly, and no longer looks at me as if I'm an idiot. "We will make all the arrangements, and I will let you know when the burial will take place."

"Thank you," your dad and I both say together, and make our way back to my pink room. Once there, we again talk desultorily. I sit on my bed, while he sits on a chair by the window. It is a large rectangular window, with a low sill. It is a sash window. My room is obviously on a corner of the brown-brick building, forming the bottom part of an L shape. I can see a garden below, with a few spindly winter trees, which seem apologetic for their existence. It is another raw day. At one stage, as our conversation subsides, I hear the same crying I heard as I was waking up that morning. It is definitely coming from the next room.

"Someone else is having a bad time," he says. Although stating the obvious, it's about the only comment that either of us feels we can make. He then tells me that all the people who've helped out looking after your brothers since I came into hospital has commented on how bright and clever they are. He says this to accentuate the positive. Your brothers are our successes. But I can see from his pale eyes that the act of saying this reminds both of us of how much they differ from you, with your damaged head and rudimentary brain. And that knowledge remains unspoken. It is still a shared secret when he leaves, to go and pick up your bright and clever brothers.

I lie on the bed for a while, undisturbed, then I hear a tap at the door. "Come in." It is Jenny, from the ante-natal class - the woman who can't bear to have her nipples touched. She looks paler, her jaw is more accentuated, and I had never noticed that she had freckles before. Now, although it is the middle of an almost sunless winter, they stand out starkly from her drained face. Her hair, in continuing to be pulled back, has taken all her colouring with it. Jenny's pale honey eyes are much smaller than I remember them, with vivid blood-red edges.

"I thought it was you, when I saw you coming into this room a little while ago," she says. "I decided to let you know I'm here too."

"What are you in for?" I ask. Despite her appearance, I deduce very little, perhaps because even the obvious is too unthinkable. I can only think that Jenny must have come in for bed rest. I did know that there had been some discrepancies between Jenny's own dates and those that a couple of recent scans had given, but I had attached no importance to it.

"I lost the baby," she suddenly sobs, and as she bursts into tears I put my arms round her and we sit down on the bed together. She weeps for a long time, and I recognise it as the same crying that I have heard coming from the next room. It must be as hard for her as it was for me to comprehend what it happening, because, between sobs, she asks me the same question.

"I lost the baby too - a little girl."

"Mine was a boy."

For the first time since you were born, I cry. I cry for Jenny, and for her dead infant, and I cry because it might appear callous not to do so. But I am dead - beyond pain - and these tears are not for you. I still can't understand that one part of me has emotionally killed me as an act of self-protection. I am aware of Jenny's despair finding vague echoes - for the moment - in a part of my being to which I have no access, and also, that I must be careful. Throughout the time I am crying, I focus only on Jenny and her baby boy. My mind continues to steer clear of my own loss. I think of the crochet hook that, less that twenty-four hours ago, broke the bag of amniotic fluid. If the crochet hook is the event, the bag of fluid is its accompanying pain. And if I am dead, they do not meet.

Many tissues later, I ask Jenny to tell me what went wrong. She says that although, in class, she told us about the discrepancies between the scans and her own dates - which, as anti-technology mothers, she knew we would dismiss anyway - she had herself sensed that the baby wasn't growing properly. This was information she had kept to herself, and worried about it. Having been detained at hospital with high blood pressure at the end of the last week, yet another scan showed that the baby had not grown for at least a few weeks. And although they had been able to detect a heartbeat early on Monday morning, the baby had died by Monday night. "It was Sister Francis who had to tell me." So - it was Jenny that Sister Francis had been thinking of, when she told me that, sometimes, she hated her job.

"What kind of delivery did you have?" I want to know to what extent Jenny's experiences have reflected mine.

"A normal induced delivery. I felt that I had failed him. The least I could do was bring him into the world. It was the only thing left that I could do for him."

There is little I can say. I can imagine nothing braver or more poignant. At the same time, I know I have not failed you. Something I am learning quickly is that I can never be other people, and that I can admire and love them and let them go. And Jenny's baby, of course, was perfect. Although both our babies are dead, we each have a different set of circumstances to come to terms with. No one is more, or less, devastating - just different.

I think back to the ante-natal classes, and the apparent physical nervousness that Jenny exhibited. All of us - including Jenny herself - had thought of her as the one who would ask for the pethidine first. I remember her funny, frantic questions: "which type of breathing?" "which type of contraction?" "which stage of labour?" "am I panting when I should be blowing?" "am I doing deep breathing when it should be shallow?"

I, along with the other members of the group, have laughed at Jenny, and she has laughed with us. Not one of us considered ever having to use the exercises to help us cope with delivering a dead baby, but Jenny has actually learnt the techniques so well that they have helped her through. I am not worthy even to know this woman, or to feel that we had anything in common. This is not because I, along with everyone else, laughed, but because, even with the benefit of two previous deliveries - for both of which I'd needed pethidine - I thought Jenny was leading the group towards something unnecessarily banal, when all I wanted was to be serious, and, I suppose, intellectual. I still craved to expand my consciousness.

Louise, I'm sorry that, had you lived, you would probably have been brought up by the person I was then, because I would not have had the experiences that changed me. If you were infinitely the most important, what I learnt from Jenny changed me completely too. She taught me about the respect due not merely to women who show courage, but to all women called on to survive the loss of a baby.

So, while the light fails
On a winters afternoon, in a secluded chapel
History is now and England.

Jenny leaves at around lunchtime. Having had her baby the day before me, she is ready to go home. Early in the afternoon, I have the first of my visitors. It is Tina, with her two youngest children. This seems somehow appropriate - having been a sentry at the last outpost as I left the outside world, she is still there as I begin to make my way back. Her hair is wilder than I remember, her cheeks and lips redder. She is wrapped in a thick black cloak and she wears black tights. She sits down in the chair by the window. She looks completely bewildered and confused. Usually so articulate, that seems to have deserted her.

"I didn't think... when I left you the other afternoon... I thought everything would be all right... I didn't think anything like that... I can't understand how it happened... I just can't believe it... Nick can't believe it either... Paul's being so brave... he's a really strong person... he's handling it so well... I couldn't believe it... it's come as such a shock... we both have such enormous respect for Paul."

"Yes, he's been brilliant. He's had to do so much organising as well," I reply, practically.

"What was the delivery like?"

"Like nothing, really. It wasn't as if I have any pain to remember. I feel okay Perhaps I'm still in shock." Tina is clearly so distressed that I feel I need to give some explanation for my apparent unconcern.

"I don't know how you can bear it," she says, and I find the implication that I have a choice somewhat bizarre. "If anything happened to me like that, I'd feel so angry."

"Maybe." I trawl the few emotions open to me, but anger is not one of them.

"I'm sorry I had to bring these two:' she tells me. "I thought the last thing you'd want to see now is healthy children, but I still felt I had to see you."

"It's not a problem," I reassure her. I do not want Tina to feel guilty. No way are these my children. I already have boys at home. Tina's baby Dominic wriggles a bit on her knee. He is now nine months old, tiny and wiry for his age, with the dark, lively eyes of a woodland animal. He stares at me from inside his winter hood. Although he looks bright and alert, he is nowhere near crawling yet. Callan props himself up against his mother, sucking his thumb. He looks suspiciously at me. I smile at him and he scowls back. I look past the matriarchal family group to the raw greyness outside.

"Thank you for looking after Benjamin and Sam," I say. "Five young kids is a hell of a handful."

"It's the only thing I felt I could do," Tina tells me. "And I've had help." Deprecating the things we, as women, actually do to help each other is pretty commonplace, and for now, I let this go. More importantly, I am starting to realise that your death has implications not just for me and your dad and your brothers, but for everyone who knows me, and that they all have to come to terms with it in their own way, perhaps by feeling emotions that I do not feel, but which are still valid for them. You touch so many lives in ways I could not have thought possible.

Our service for you is to take place at half past three. Your dad comes in soon after three. We hug each other, and he updates me on your brothers, who are still fine, and says that he will bring them to see me again in the evening. Then there is a knock on the door. It is Michael. He has come to take the service, but wanted to see us beforehand.

"Oh Penny." He holds out his arms to me. "I'm so very, very sorry."

"Michael." Suddenly, this man, dressed in his simple black clerical clothes, holding out his arms to me in quiet dignity, calls from my soul all I have lost and gives it an incomprehensible power to hurt me. I cry violently, from somewhere in my stomach that is being torn apart. And even while I am crying, looking down, I see that even this is little compared with what is to come: that pain reaches into uncharted parts of my psyche and my being, where you are, yet you are not. And despite feeling Michael's arms round me, I know that, ultimately, in going through it, I will be alone. But I also know that, somehow, I will come through.

As my mind returns again to the pink room, I see that your dad too has been crying, and I move away from Michael, who goes to prepare for the service, and put my arms round him. Then two midwifery sisters arrive from the ward. Middle-aged and kind-looking, they are going to come to the chapel with us. Your dad and I sort ourselves out. This is your service, and we want to remember it clearly, rather than through a haze of emotion that we can give vent to later.

"Ready to face it?" he asks gently.

"Ready." My reply is small but resolute.

It is the third service of its kind he has been to with me. First my mum, five-and-a half years ago, in high summer, then my dad, two months after that, now you. I can't help thinking that his life might have been less traumatic without me.

Oh my love. Perhaps there are more beautiful services, but I shall never be privileged again to attend one. Whatever spirit God is, walks here, on this December afternoon. The two midwives follow behind, and your dad and I hold hands as we enter the chapel. Michael is already at the front, in his vestments, and you are there too, before the altar, in a hospital perspex crib. Above the altar, there are stained glass windows. Like the chapel itself, they are small and perfect. You look asleep, but too peaceful even for that. That serenity you brought to my life last night, when I first saw your face, is still there. This time, you are wrapped all in pink, your little head covered with a pink blanket. Your mouth is still open. My daughter.

Michael stands beside your crib. He reads simply, from a prayer book, letting the words speak for themselves. He seems to have recognised that your dad and I would prefer the words of the old liturgy, with their resonance. He blesses you. He also makes some references to God and Jesus, which wash over me. Even for your sake, at the moment, I cannot embrace Christianity. But he does say something about not understanding why things happen, and all we can do is hope that we can accept them, and I find that true. I look at you, and in your calmness, know that you have accepted that you could not come to me, your brothers or your dad - at least, not in this life.

There are only six of us in the little chapel, and, while Michael has been speaking, it has grown dark outside. There is no colour now in the stained-glass windows, and the light at the front of the chapel shines only on us. We are together in this pool of light, in our grief and yet joined somehow, in a sense of wonder. Michael invites us to pray silently together for a few minutes, and I do this, kneeling down but looking at you, absorbing every detail of your lovely face. There is nothing I can pray for - I have already lost everything - but there is contemplation, and I know the infinite touches us all that afternoon, and that we are held eternally, and that you have taken us out of time.

Slowly, we come back to the moment, and Michael indicates that the service is over.

"May I say goodbye?" I ask, as quietly as I can.

"Of course." Your dad and I approach the altar. I know this is the last time I will ever see you. I gaze at your face again, at your blanket. Again, I am ready to let you go - this time, forever. I brush your cheek with my hand.

"Goodbye my love." I am unaware of how I feel, but it is hard to speak, and two tears fall unexpectedly onto your blanket.

The midwives are waiting at the back of the chapel, ready to take us back. Despite their years of experience, they too have been crying, but they are there for our support. One puts her arm round my waist, and the other does the same to your dad. That way, we are taken back to the ward.

When we get there, we discover that Rosie is already in the room. She'd been told where we were, and had decided to wait for us. I start to tell her about the service, but before I can, it's your dad's turn to be hit with what we have lost. He sits over by the window, crying relentlessly. Then as I move towards him, he stands up, so I can hold him better.

"She would have been so lovely, so lovely, he sobs." I hold him tight, and notice Rosie looking questioningly at me. I nod. She comes over and holds the two of us. I cry again - for you, for me, for your dad. Yes, you would have been - are - so lovely. We stay like that for several minutes.

Then your dad, with an effort, stops crying and, characteristically, resumes sorting out practical things. He has to collect your brothers from Alison's and give them their tea. He puts on his Home's overcoat, jerking the belt tight, as if that will fasten in all the hurt he is feeling, and reminds me that he will bring Benjamin and Sam back to see me.

When we are alone, Rosie and I have another cuddle.

"I felt that she was a baby for all of us," I whisper. "A daughter for our future."

"I know," Rosie reassures me, "we all thought that."

"At least," I exclaim with sudden vehemence, "I'll never have to worry about her being killed in a nuclear attack, will I?"

"That's true." Rosie looks at me doubtfully. It is a savage form of comfort.

Looking from a window above
It's like a story of love
Can you hear me?
Came back only yesterday
Moving further away
Want you near me

Shortly before tea, I have another visitor. It is Beth, from the ante-natal class, whose shoulders I massaged, getting ready to have you. Last night, there was an ante-natal class, and Jayne had to tell the other women what had happened to both Jenny and me. In fact, at the same time that the other women in the group were practising their panting and blowing and having their backs rubbed, you had just been born, both deaths casting a shadow into every corner of the evening. It occurs to me that Jayne will have been the first person to find out about both - first, a call from Bjorn, and, while still coming to terms with that blow, a call from your dad, a day later. Because of our complications, Jenny and I have produced the first babies in Jayne's first class since qualifying. Dead babies.

"I wanted to come and see you as soon as I could," Beth tells me. We hug each other, and I find reassurance in the softness of her body, and of her voice, which floats on an undercurrent of breath.

"None of us can really believe it," she continues. "It hasn't sunk in yet. Please let me know if there's anything any of us can do to help."

I say that I will, and sink back onto the bed, resting on propped-up pillows. Beth perches on the bed. Her hair has the same cut but it now seems dark red rather than plum - nearly the same colour as Jenny's. She is wearing a voluminous pale grey, tweedy coat - well, more of a cloak, really, with slits for her hands to go through. She is obviously heavily pregnant, but to me, it doesn't matter. Beth shifts somewhat uncomfortably, though, as if she perceives her bulk as a reminder of a living child to come, and that's what I don't have any more. If that's what she does feel, I admire and love her even more for coming. And as I am still somewhere between elation and emotional death, I find it easy to convince her - as I have convinced myself - that everything's okay and that although you are dead, I can cope with it and the experience of having had you is enough.

"She is still my daughter," I explain. "And I know I will never lose sight of that, no matter what happens."

Beth smiles myopically at me from behind her round glasses.

"You're being very brave," she remarks encouragingly. I don't contradict her, but think that I haven't really had anything to be brave about. She asks after your brothers, and your dad, and I tell her how they have taken it. And as she kisses me and leaves, I realise how much better she is at this than I ever was, before it happened to me. She didn't mind being with me, she never worried about not saying the right thing, or saying something inadequate. She understood instinctively that being there for someone is what matters, even if you haven't had their experience yourself.

The next person who visits looks just as confused and bewildered as Tina. His hair is wilder too, than I remember. It is Dr Walker. Throughout all his experience of delivering babies and doing post and ante-natal checks, he has had only one other patient who had an anencephalic baby.

"Were the symptoms similar to mine?"

"Yes, I suppose they were. But the baby could have just been breech, and as you said yourself, you carry a lot of fluid in your pregnancies. I could never have thought that it would happen twice, within a year, in the same practice."

I feel quite sorry for him. I imagine he feels that he has been dumped on from a great height. He believes in what he does, he believes in a woman's right to have her babies how she wants them. He is the only doctor in the town prepared to undertake home deliveries, to encourage natural childbirth and to avoid unnecessary medical interference. He knows how important these were to me, because I sought him out in the first place, and from the conversations we have had since. We are both on the side of life. He, and Sister Lennox, are the people in the medical profession who know exactly how much I've lost in that respect.

I give him an account, not only of the scan and delivery, and how my feelings about you have changed, and he begins to brighten. But he does have one last question.

"Would it have helped if you'd had a scan?" And of course, I've thought about that one as well.

"No. When I found out, I thought it would, but at least this way, I have had a baby."

The corners of Dr Walker's thin mouth turn upwards in a grin. There is a knock at the door. It's Jayne. She has had her hair highlighted and she's wearing a deliciously pink lipstick. As she smiles, the familiar dimples appear on her cheeks. She gives me a hug and sits down on the bed, opposite Dr Walker.

"Hi." They exchange greetings. She has seen him more since qualifying as an NCT teacher, and, of course, she has put quite a lot of business his way. I also remember that he was her GP when she lost her twins. He has been here before.

"How are you?" As Jayne addresses me, I hear the concern in her voice. There is no great chasm separating Jayne and me, as there has now been between me and all my other visitors. Between us, we have lost three daughters. Jayne has been where I am now, and although I wouldn't wish this on anyone else, I am so relieved to meet someone else to whom this happened - and who survived it. But it is Dr Walker who replies to her question.

"I expected to be really depressed, but Penny's really cheered me up."

"Really?" Jayne turns to me, her eyebrows arched. She doesn't seem to believe it.

"Yes" Dr Walker gives a brief resume of my positive attitude, and says that he's really glad he came, and he'll look forward to seeing me at home now.

"I'm glad you feel okay" Jayne informs me. "I hope it lasts." Her painfully blue eyes are full of doubt. The dimples have gone from her cheeks.

"It was a very subdued evening at yesterday's class," she continues. "With you and Jenny, it was too much for us really to take in. Everyone is devastated for both of you. So very, very sorry. They all send their love."

"Thanks", I reply, somewhat wistfully. For the second time today, I am grateful for their thoughts, but I wonder how many of them now worry that they might lose their babies, like Jenny and I have done.

Jayne is now deflected from her thoughts about me by a direct question from Dr Walker.

"How many weeks is it now? Are you still feeling all right, or have you had any sickness so far?"

I don't think have ever seen Jayne go red before. A flush begins just below her neck and spreads right over her forehead. She looks at Dr Walker for a fraction of a second, and then down at my bedcover.

"Yes, yes," she whispers to the cover. "Everything's fine." Dr Walker looks at Jayne, grinning. I look bemused. Suddenly, Jayne turns her eyes full on me. "I'm pregnant," she says, "but please keep it to yourself for a while. It's only eight weeks, so I've a long time to go. And 'many a slip 'twixt cup and lip', as they say."

The metaphor conjures up a graphic image in my mind of cups and lips, much more than the idea of a baby, and somehow gets mixed up with it. Of course, Dr Walker has not been privy to this idea of Jayne's that she would keep the pregnancy secret until later, so I unexpectedly get to know. As Jayne was to remark some time later, "I was rather sorry that you found out that way. That evening was about you, really."

I look at Jayne, as if, by so doing, I can work out how I feel, because I do not altogether like it. I know there is a sense of envy in me that was missing when Beth came to see me. Why? God knows, if anyone deserves this, it's Jayne. Please don't let me feel anything but happy for her. But I did not know of Jayne's pregnancy before I had you, and that is the difference. In some obscure way, even this feels like a betrayal - as will every pregnancy I hear about for a long time to come. I also realise that Jayne has got to a point where she feels able to try again - that she has put a distance of grief between her daughters and her new baby, so that she will be able to love the newcomer in his or her own right, rather than as a substitute Emily or Claire. And I want to be in Jayne's position, having gone through what I glimpsed today when Michael held me in his arms, and not to have it to come. Silently, I ask to be forgiven for my selfishness, and for Jayne's baby to be healthy and happy.

After they have both gone, I have a little time to myself, before your dad brings your brothers round. It is quite a late night for them. Sam disappears under the bed for most of the visit, while Benjamin chats for a bit then does his own bit of exploring round the room. They seem to take everything - the loss of the baby, their mum not being around and having to be in hospital - just as something that's happened. Apparently, it doesn't involve their emotions at all.

And they scarcely involve mine. I know that I should be grateful to have these two healthy children, and in my head, I can hear a future echo from misinformed well-wishers - "well, at least you've got Benjamin and Sam." Still largely detached from my emotions, I know, to a deep part of my mind, that no amount of healthy children will ever make up for the loss of this one. And the trauma of having you has robbed me of the ability to feel anything, at the moment, for anyone previously close to me. I know that I do still love them and that I couldn't bear to lose them, but they have lost their capacity to affect me. They are beautiful objects, trapped behind a glass case. I want to understand why I have been allowed to have these two children and not my daughter, and whether God has been involved in some kind of trade-off. "You can't have the daughter you wanted, but I have these top-of-the-range male versions. Attractive, responsible children with very clever minds. What's that? No, I'm sorry, it's not negotiable. Take it or leave it."

Benjamin looks briefly at me with his big blue eyes, then takes an interest in the photo of you that's on my bedside table. I tell him that is his sister, but she was already dead when the photo was taken. He looks at it solemnly, then goes for another wander. Sam emerges from underneath the bed.

I kiss them goodnight, unconvincingly. I don't want them to be damaged- I have a prescience of how much I will come to care for them again - but, like the name Rebecca, I would like them to be wrapped in tissue paper and safely stored in a drawer labelled "life," until I am ready for them again.

Later, the ancillary bringing my night-time drink notices something of a puddle under the bed. It must have been Sam. We are going through a phase where it isn't worth putting him back in nappies, but he is quite often damp around what Alison calls the nether regions. As she leaves to fetch a mop, a fluttering of something half-remembered brushes across my mind. It's something I once called love.

Love is itself unmoving,
only the cause and end of movement...
Caught in the form of limitation
Between un-being and being.

When I wake up the next morning, I feel as if I have come out of a coma. I have no memory of my dreams, but they have taken me immense distances while my body was lead-heavy and did not move. I know immediately what I still have to face, and I come round slowly, keeping my body still for a long time. I really do not want to wake up. But today, I am going home, and I must be ready.

I wash automatically, scrutinising my face again in the mirror for clues to explain this to me, but the same rounded, ripe features blankly return my gaze. I get dressed fragilely. I pack my few belongings, gathering the two photos and the birth card from my bedside table last of all, and reverently placing them at the top of the bag. Now there is nothing to do, so I lie on my bed and watch the black-and-white portable TV that I was presented with on the first evening. They are showing some repeats of My Music, which I used to watch quite a lot with my own mum and dad, and then later, with your dad. At the end of the programme, Steve Race always gets each of the panellists to sing. This time, he asks Ian Wallace to sing a song I've never heard before or since, but a phrase from its chorus haunts me still, as you do. The song is about a sailor who has to leave someone behind just as a relationship is developing, and he tells the woman involved:

And I would have loved you so, my dear,
I would have loved you so.

And for the second time since your birth, it's something achingly simple that cracks the shell of unfeeling, that twists my stomach in a physical pain and forces me to see, if not begin to comprehend, what I have lost. So much love. Oh my darling. I might have begun by wanting you for the wrong reasons, I may have pretended and played different parts, but this is the truth. For as long as I live, my love for you will be the most honest part of my life imaginable.

What happens to it now? It was there, a jar inside me that had been gradually filling throughout the pregnancy, as you grew and developed within me. It started from such unpromising beginnings - I want her, I don't want her, I want her, I don't want her - that pendulum swinging in its confusion of the unsure and selfish person I was then. But even then, a few scarce drops of a pure essence found their way into the jar, and as I accepted the inevitable, defended us against your dad's unwanting, felt you move, and carried you almost to the end of the forty weeks, that jar had been filled to the brim, ready for all that love to spill over you when you came to me. Maybe who I was then was not very much to give you, Louise, but it was a genuine mother's love, and despite those bad beginnings, you would have been so welcome in our family. I know my love for you might not have been perfect, but it was real, and it is what I had ready to give you. And you will never know. And as I cry into the comfortless pillow, the question returns - what happens to it now? How can I give it to you, when you are not here? How can it change, grow, develop - if you can't? Is it simply transposed into grief for a lost life?

Or will it simply leak away, un-saveable? I waited so long for you to come to me - I waited, with so much love to give - all now lost. I cry for a long, long time.

> *And I would have loved you so, my dear,*
> *I would have loved you so.*

Later, I have my last two visitors - Sister Lennox, and the Health Visitor from the practice, Mrs. Marchant. I vaguely know Mrs. Marchant, who has visited the flat a couple of times to check on your brothers' development and who, I gather, has now become something of an expert in diet and health. This is the early eighties, and there is a lot of money to be made by people in this field. As I find out later, Mrs. Marchant is using her practice experience to build up a future clientele for when she sets up on her own. She is, I reckon, in her early fifties. Her greying hair is swept back from a smooth, broad forehead. Everything about her is plain but expensive - she lets quality speak for itself. Her suit and blouse are grey, her earrings are gold. Her engagement ring is a single, perfect diamond that catches the fluorescent light and breaks into a myriad of colours. Her veined hands have tapering fingers and well-manicured nails. She reminds me of a head teacher. Sister Lennox looks very upset, asks if I've seen Jayne, and says that she will be looking after me. She looks rather uncomfortable and out of place, and I get the impression she will be happier to see me at home. I remember that, after all, the medical profession still needs to treat me as if I've had a baby. She asks if I've seen Jayne, and looks relieved when I tell her I have. Then it's Mrs. Marchant's turn. There is a hard edge to her voice as she says she's sorry for what happened. Then she asks quite bluntly,

"Do you think there may have been anything wrong with your diet around the time of conception?"

You're not even in your grave yet, I'm still in the hospital where I had you, and I am being asked this. I want to think and talk about you, if I want to talk at all. I certainly don't want to explore putative explanations with someone I hardly know. I am developing my own interests in diet and health - soon to become something of an obsession - but this is simply not what I want to discuss, and think it crass of Mrs. Marchant to have come to the hospital purely to hawk her own interests because of my distress.

"No, I don't think so. I'm sure I have a more than adequate diet."

"Yes, you probably do think that." Mrs. Marchant smoothes creases from her grey skirt. "But it certainly wouldn't hurt to have an expert opinion."

"Perhaps I'll come and see you another time then. Not now." Before, I had hoped to have provided a curt enough reply for her not to continue the conversation. This time, I do seem to have succeeded. I know that deeply, I am confused and hurting, but at the same time, certain things have acquired a strange lucidity. Losing my baby does not give this woman - even if she is a health visitor - the right to make me part of her personal crusade and for once in my life, I will have the temerity to tell her so. At the same time, there is a thought, around diet and responsibility for your condition, that I do not want to face yet. I do not articulate it, and put it on a high dusty shelf in my mind.

Later, while I am waiting for Jayne to come and take me home, another nurse comes in to check my blood pressure, then reprimands me for sitting with my legs crossed. I uncross them, and resist the temptation to tell this woman to sort her priorities out when dealing with a mother who's just lost a baby. I may have baulked one medical professional that morning, but I do not yet have the confidence to keep it up.

Jayne has kindly offered to give me a lift back to the flat. She arrives punctually at half past eleven. She even carries my few possessions to the car. I have not been outside for nearly three days. The weather is still grittily grey, the air is dirty with winter, mainly still, but there is some wind, carried on the sea's bite. We drive the short distance to Chapel Park Road, along wide roads lined with rambling - and in some cases crumbling - Victorian houses, now mainly broken up into flats and bedsits. Neglected, they are the sad legacy of many broken dreams. Even from the car, I notice pile after pile of dog mess on the pavements.

"Do you want me to come in?" Jayne asks supportively, as we pull up. Then, as I hesitate, she adds, "or would you rather be in the bosom of your family?" No, I wouldn't rather, but it's what I sense we somehow ought to do. I express my thanks to Jayne for the lift and for all her support, but fail to find the words to thank her for being so perceptive. Yes, I do want her to come in, I want to keep this link with the only other woman I really know who has stood where my soul now stands, but I know that first, your dad, your brothers and I must be reunited as a family unit. Jayne and I hug, and I get out of the car. As I walk towards the door, Jayne drives away.

Of all the different sorts of pain involved in losing a baby, coming home with empty arms has got to be one of the worst single moments. A healthy baby fills so much more than a mother's arms - her whole being and her home resonate with the amazing power of new life. But when she goes away to have a baby and comes back with - with nothing, just an absence: the emptiness of her arms expands and pours into every corner of her being and her home. Because of nothing, there is only the most intense pain of loss imaginable. I want to hold my arms out to something, to fill them up, to fill up my being, my home with anything, anything, but there is nothing I know, nothing I love, that can in any way ever be adequate - not your dad, not your brothers, not even another baby. Only you. Only holding you in my arms could heal, could make the flat seem smaller. I can reach others, I know they are there for me. But even holding those I love is a cruel travesty of holding you. I reach out for comfort, for I do not have you. You are the reference-point. You live in and between everyone I thought I could get close to. And while I may reach out for comfort, could I ever again reach out for joy?

I walk a long lonely way through the hall, with these thoughts, then I open the door to the front room, where your dad and your brothers are playing, but they are so subdued it is like watching them on T.V. with the sound turned down. Since leaving Jayne, I have been too overwhelmed to cry. Then your dad, who has obviously been crying recently, simply takes my hand and leads me over to the dresser. He has had to perform the awful task of telling so many people, and already, we know our grief is shared. The dresser is festooned with flowers - including some from Lesley's family in Brighton, who still live near my parents' old flat. The others are from people in your dad's office, and Hastings NCT. He has placed the cards on the dresser. I pick them up, fingering each one in turn.

"People are very kind," he says, and that is enough. The thought of kindness triggers both our tears. We stand together crying for quite a long time, holding each other tightly, totally united in our grief. The boys look up at us, then come and put their little arms around our knees. When your dad and I are calmer, we put your photo and your birth card with the flowers. We have made a little shrine to you.

From now on, whenever we have visitors, one of your brothers will take it in turns to take them over to the dresser, show them the photo and tell them,

"That's Mummy and Daddy with the baby. The baby died, and it's poorly there." It's as if they'd rehearsed it together.

Already, there is post to open. Your dad rang Sylvia as soon as you were born, and the news has already reached Olivia. She has written straight away - on a card with doves on the front. There is also a letter from your dad's uncle - your great-uncle. In many ways, they epitomise the two types of letter we received. I will let both letters speak for themselves, to end this chapter.

Thursday

To you both,

I'm so sorry and sad for you. All the love and hopes that you invest in a pregnancy, the nicknames you give the baby, the joy you feel when it kicks, and that lovely Cheshire cat feeling - the "I'm growing a baby," are so special and extraordinary, that I can only cry with frustration and anger when it comes to nothing. Life is so precious. I'm sorry Louise couldn't fulfil all the dreams and wishes you must have had for her.

I can imagine that the scan and the trip for X-rays, then the induction must have been like being flung into the vortex of a nightmare - the one thing you can never believe in, happening to you. Poor Penny - I know that path too well, although Rowan, Amber and I cheated death by a hair's breadth. If only I could give you a huge hug. I know that nothing ever takes the place of a stillborn child. My mum had one - her first child - and all thro' my life, even tho' I never knew her, she had a special place in the family. It was nice, not spooky. Mum was very bitter that she'd not been allowed to hold her: I'm glad you held Louise and have a photo of her.

The possibility of an MA in Women in Education sounds exciting, much better than being stuck in the sticks of Stainton! It'll give you much food for thought, but don't let it take the place of grief. Perhaps we are too advanced a civilisation and grief is pushed into the background as unseemly. I hope you'll have lots of support, people who'll spend time talking, crying and mourning with you. Dear Penny, I do wish I could come and cuddle you. It would be an awfully wet meeting because I can't stop crying for you. Instead, here are some Doves - for the Peace you'll need now.

With very much love, Olivia.
love too, at Christmas and Peace for 1984

P.S. You must be prepared for the rats who will try to make you feel guilty because you'd arranged a home delivery - a form of 'I told you so.' Hateful people and you'll need strength to deal with them. I believe in Fate, pre-ordination somehow. You'll find out the reason later in your life, but needn't look for it now.

Chesterfield
14.12.83

To you all,
We have just talked to Mum on the phone and thought we should write at once to say we share your sorrow and distress. For all your plans to have reached this stage and then for this to happen is a terrible blow. From last night when we had the first news we felt sick and although it couldn't have altered the final outcome it ought to have been possible to have a scan at an earlier stage. I hope if I say we have to carry on it doesn't sound hard or matter-of-fact. I certainly don't mean it to but no matter what happens we do have to carry on. This is not to say that an experience like you have just had will not make its mark or indeed help us all to learn some lesson. On the bright side you have the boys and they will continue to give great pleasure. This is not intended to be a newsy letter but just to assure you that you are in our thoughts and we shall look forward to seeing you soon.

Yours,
Uncle Doug and Auntie June

This is gonna take a long time
And I wonder what's mine
Can't take no more
Wonder if you understand
It's just the touch of your hand
Behind a closed door

It takes your dad and I a little while to assimilate the contents of both letters. We are walking around with constant aches at the centre of our beings. I want to keep a fence around us but your brothers' needs make that impossible. Yet your dad seems to welcome their noise, their hunger, their thirst, their runny noses, their frequent visits to the toilet - all the things that make life with young children normal. And I am happy for him to take over, while I try to stare into the middle distance and into silence. But I feel as if I am constantly interrupted, and that their abundance of life is doing nothing but bruising my grief.

So I feel relieved when your dad takes them to the St. Andrew's Toddler Group Christmas party. He is going into work for the afternoon, and they will be looked after, then brought home, by Alison and Tina. I think that, once they have gone, it will be like being in the hospital. I think it will give me the chance to be alone with my grief. But almost as soon as the door closes behind them, and I hear their little voices receding up the road, I realise it is not the same. This is my home, this is where those dearest to me live, this is where you should be. This is mainly where you have lived for the last nine months. It's where you should have come back to. I cannot bear the emptiness, the resounding silence. The flat is hideously vast, and bizarre as anything Alice encountered in wonderland.

Sobbing, I walk around the flat. I peer into most of the rooms, as if somehow, if I only look hard enough, I will find you. For in a sense, I am wrong. It's not the emptiness that's as awful as the lacerating sense of your presence. I find myself pulling back bed covers, looking in the airing cupboard - even lifting the lid of the freezer. You live everywhere, in every room. You are everywhere, yet you are nowhere. I am frightened of the pain. I don't know how I can bear it.

Finally, I open the door of my bedroom very deliberately and go in, closing it softly behind me. I was last in here before I went to Sussex for my interview. I share this bedroom with your dad, and because the flat has only two bedrooms, we were to share it with you - at least, while you were a little baby. In the hospital, he had asked me whether I wanted him to remove all the things we had got ready for you.

"No," I told him. "I will still know what you have done, and the artificiality will be as bad as any reminders."

Everything is still as I left it - things for you, things for the home delivery. Two corners of the large bedroom are dedicated to you. Your cot - the one your dad got from work, which we never did get round to painting - is there in one corner. Inside it is a Moses basket, a pile of babygrows, some stabbingly tiny vests and some little cardigans. Your pram - a chocolate-colour carry cot on wheels - is in the other corner, and it contains all that brown paper. I pick up one of the vests, holding it to my face. It smells freshly washed, and soon it is soaked with my tears. You will never wear it.

This, more than anywhere else that will ever be, is where you are, and yet you are not. Here, I could reach out my hand, touch your living flesh. Oh God. Under the crushing weight of pain, I sink to my knees, at the same time, suddenly crying out, wailing more loudly than I could have imagined possible. I, who normally cry so discreetly, shriek, and scream into the empty air. I am screaming from somewhere so deep inside me it tears me in two.

"Why?" I shout several times, each scream stronger than the last, as though that might bring an answer. "No, no, no, please, no." I scream that too, holding onto the bars of the cot for support. This is a primal, prostrating, noisy, incoherent grief. This desperate futile wailing is the only way I can meet it. I am facing the rest of my life.

I don't care who hears me. I have a right to cry like this, to disturb the universe. I want my voice, my only expression of a sorrow so great I don't know how I can bear it, to be carried through the walls, through the trees, through the sea, out, out, through time and space, to all I can comprehend of eternity and infinity. For surely you must be somewhere? Is it possible that I could search forever and never find you? Or must I die to be with you? Is that what it takes? If I die, my darling, will you come to me? Oh my love. My dearest love. I want nothing more. How can I make it happen?

I am crying more normally now, and the storm is subsiding. I am lying on the floor, in a foetal position, drained and exhausted, still clutching your little vest. I don't know how long I have been there before I hear the doorbell. Thank God. I need other people right now. With wobbly legs, I get up. Slowly I make my way through our hallway and through the high, echoing, white communal hall to the front door of the house.

It is Sue Marriott. Her brown wiry hair too looks uncombed. There is a halo of mist round its edges. She starts to cry as soon as she sees me, and I haven't really finished. She holds out a little posy of flowers.

"These are all that my garden can produce at the moment." They are damply bedraggled, their purple and yellow heads bowed but brave. Sue puts her arm round me and supports me as we go into the front room. I place the little flowers on the dresser, and make them part of the shrine.

"I'm so sorry, Penny, so sorry. This is the worst thing that could happen."

"Yes," I tell her between sniffs, "it is. I know that now." I hardly know Sue, but your death gives us a sudden intimacy that otherwise would have taken years to develop. I tell Sue about what has just happened, including my somewhat unhinged wanderings through the flat, and show her your creased and tear-drenched vest. I talk her through everything - the delivery, the dog doctor, the service. She simply holds my hands between hers and listens and listens. She allows me plenty of time for silence, and plenty of time for tears. She sheds her own from time to time, in quiet dignity. By the time I finish, and offer her tea, it is getting dark. I get up and close the curtains and switch on the light. As I go out to the kitchen, I realise I actually feel better. I feel you even closer to me, but it is a closeness that comforts rather than threatening to destroy. I feel more uplifted than I could have imagined when I was alone in the flat, just for talking with a woman who loves me. Even our spacious front room looks comparatively cosy when I return with the tea. I could never really explain to Sue that in some way, she has saved my life.

We drink from the reindeer mugs. The unicorn has now vanished forever, but it wasn't me who killed it. I cup my hands round the warm pottery.

"I brought something else," Sue says. I open another dove card - this time, a hand-made one of a stunningly white dove, with a pattern of leaves, of greens and browns, around the edge. Inside, in calligraphy, it simply says,

I place that, too, on the shrine, next to Olivia's dove card. Symbol of peace. Alison and Tina return your brothers from the toddler group party soon after Sue leaves, and this time, I am much more welcoming. Tina is also accompanied by her three children, so we have quite a houseful. Sam is wearing different dungarees - it has all been too exciting for him. Joyously, both he and Benjamin show me the toys they have been given by Santa. Their eyes sparkle with happiness, and we share our first real moment of contact since I lost you. Christmas is starting to have a fresh meaning now that I have young children. Despite myself, every year I love to play my part in creating with them the magic of Christmas. I feel a pang of anguish to realise that you will never share this with us, or the cynicism that comes with growing up, but for now, I am in control of the pain, and can live with what I have. Yet when your dad returns from work, and the flat is empty of visitors, and he offers to put your brothers to bed, I let him. I cannot yet tackle the practical burden. I feel a headache coming on and go and lie down on our low bed. Light hurts, but I do not want to be alone in the darkness. I leave the door open and a slice of light from the hallway outside falls over the floor and onto my legs.

A bit later, after your brothers are in bed, I call out to your dad that I can see flashing lights in front of my left eye. I am a bit panicky because I don't know what it is, and he rings Dr Walker. This is, apparently, a migraine. I am surprised. The flashing lights are putting on a good display, but the pain is not as incapacitating as I believe migraine pain can be. I've had worse headaches, but never these flashing lights before, so I imagine this must be my first ever migraine. I wonder about the epidural. But even if this is cause and effect, it seems that one more totally new and bizarre experience will not make a lot of difference around here.

I have one more visitor. It is Sharon Clayton, the woman from St. Andrew's toddler group who lent me, in all innocence, the set of maternity clothes containing that unlucky pinafore dress. She only found out what has happened at the Christmas party that afternoon. Your dad asks if it's okay for her to visit. I ask her not to stay long, on account of my headache. She lowers herself to sit on the bed beside me, still wearing her black leather coat. I don't invite her to take it off. I now remember Sharon telling me about twins she had when she was very young - no more than seventeen. A boy and a girl, they had died, like Jayne's twins, and Helen Jones' Joshua, through being born too early. At the time, she had promised herself that she would never have any more children. Six years later she got drunk one Christmas, and Sarah, who had been three in September, was the result. She also now had Jasmin, now one, but had nearly miscarried with her.

"So I'm quitting while I'm still ahead," she had told me one Friday afternoon. At this moment, in the half-light, through the jagged lights in my left eye, I can see that her very long dark hair is pulled away from her face. It cascades down her back. She can almost sit on it. Sharon has very narrow eyes - think they are green - but I see they are trained on me now, searching my face in concern. I tell her too about the delivery - about holding you - and I notice that each telling is getting easier. Certain phrases are repeated, so each telling is, in a sense, a rehearsal for the next one. This is our story Louise, and through being spread, in the same language, it becomes more immutably so. Through telling it, I get to keep it as it hardens, becoming something almost as tangible as your photo and your birth card. A telling and a keeping. I also notice that the better I know the words of the events, the less power those events have to wound, when I describe them to others. And that too is a form of healing.

I also tell Sharon about the Ian Wallace song

And l would have loved you so, my dear,
I would have loved you so.

"Not would have, Penny," she says, "do. You do love her."

"Yes, I do - but what happens to it?" Sharon looks as if she does not understand what I am saying. Perhaps the question is unanswerable.

"As soon as I heard," Sharon goes on, "it brought it all back. It was as if all the years in between haven't happened at all, and I thought, 'I must go to Penny and be with her.'"

"Thanks." I smile at Sharon and her thickish lips smile back at me. Then realise that she has come as much for her own sake as for mine, although she would not have meant it that unkindly. She was so tenderly young when it happened to her.

"Tell me about your babies," I ask Sharon, as gently as I can.

So she does. Donna and Luke, she called them. Luke was very tiny and died almost immediately. Donna was rather more robust, and lived for about a day. She goes into graphic descriptions of them, of the delivery. She tells me how she hardly knows what happened in the two years after they were born. It was as if she went to sleep for that time, then suddenly woke up and found out she had a husband, a home and a life to get on with. She was only nineteen.

So that's how people who lost babies go on living, I think. Not necessarily by going into depression, or even going mad - although I can visualise either - or both - happening to me if this afternoon is anything to go by; but rather somehow, something that passes for life comes along and shovels layers and layers of other experiences on top. Some are more meaningful than others. Some may even fool you for a time that they matter. But it's there, always there, buried at the centre, waiting, waiting, to burst through again in all its crippling lacerating rawness. And one of the most potent triggers is the birth, known to you, of a dead baby.

After she has told her story, Sharon takes my hand. And then we are a motionless tableau. I don't know how long we remain like that. The only sense of movement I feel is centred at the left side of my left eye, where the lights continue their jagged flashing, and a feeling of seasickness in my stomach. From the outside, we are still.

And it is with little motion that Sharon departs. She gives my hand a gentle squeeze and asks to be told when the funeral is. She is a short woman, yet her black leather coat and black glossy hair seem to glide from the room.

I know that she has seen herself out. I am also becoming increasingly aware that, although many good wishes are being sent to us, they are nearly all from my friends, and that your dad does not have the same network of support that I do. Keeping my head as still as I can, I go and join him in the front room, where he is watching some aimless programme on the television. I sit down in front of him, and put my head on his lap. Even if I can't do much on a practical level, there is some emotional support I can offer. We are still. We are together. Still. Together.

Then suddenly, we jump apart at the shrill ring of the telephone. It's Olivia. She and I talk for a long time, although she largely repeats the content of her card. I know I am muted, even for the situation. I want the contact, yes - but what I really want right now is silent sharing - and the phone does not permit that. Eventually I put the phone down and go back to your dad, still waiting patiently in the same position. This time, we decide to go to bed, although it's still early,

and ignore any further interruptions. It is the first night in many months that we have been able
to have a really close cuddle. For you are no longer between us, in any sense, and now, you
never will be.

So I find words I never thought to speak
In streets I never thought I should revisit
When I left my body on a distant shore.

The darkness can be more easily felt than you. We cling to each other, unmoving, in the
palpable darkness.
Then, from the basement below comes the sound of tuneless music, played on what
sounds like a Hammond organ.
"What the hell's that?" I ask, breaking the pattern of our own stillness. "It's Irene,
downstairs. She started last night."
"It sounds like crematorium music," I realise there is the bubble of a giggle in my tummy.
"I know." I can hear your dad's voice has the edge of a laugh to it too. "I'm not sure if it's
coincidence or if it's being done for our benefit."
We never did find out - it was not the sort of thing that was easy to ascertain. I just
remember that, from suppressed giggles, our laughter mounted and mounted, disturbing the
thick darkness, until the music stopped, and we were drained again of emotion. Farce in the
midst of tragedy. The light relief of the ridiculous.

32 Family Values

Time past and time future
What might have been and what has been
Point to one end, which is always present.

When I try to wake up the next morning, I know I don't want to. It's much more than facing waking up without you, as I now know I will have to do every day for the rest of my life. It's also more than waking up with the muzziness around my head which is the aftermath of my migraine. I have now to do my own share of the phone calls - the less pressing, but still important calls to family who are not close, but who still need to be told. People who have known me all my life, to whom I am related by blood, but whom I would never have chosen as my friends. Most of their values and political beliefs are diametrically opposed to mine.

Added to that, whenever I think of them, I involuntarily remember my primary and early secondary years, when my mother proudly paraded my school reports and other academic achievements at every family gathering - Christmas, Easter and August Bank Holiday. Later, at school itself, I learnt to become quite adept at hiding my ability, having discovered that it set me apart and made me unpopular, and I imagined that it had had that effect on my extended family. Added to that, I had been set up, in my aspirant working-class nuclear family, as the Clever One, the one who would Achieve Things. It had been a grievous blow to my mother when I had turned my back on an academic career and gone into teaching, partly because she bought I was underachieving and would be unfulfilled – and in that, I think, she turned out to be right - but also because it appeared to those to whom she had lauded my talents and abilities that I had failed to realise my potential. My ability gave her a long overdue sense of value -and, it must be said, of superiority - among her friends and family, and I took it away from her. I don't think she ever really accepted it.

If we could meet now, in some soft blue twilight place which is neither life nor death, I would want her to know how right she was. Rejecting one path because you fear it will suffocate you does not necessarily mean that its alternative will, in the long term, be any more fulfilling - only different. Both of us were wrong - both of us were right. My daughter, this is a truth I would pass on to you, if you and I could only meet, just briefly, in that same soft place.

Yet while I had deliberately rejected socially conventional markers of success, I felt vulnerable before my extended family, in not achieving something I had set out to do. And that, I have to admit to you, Louise, was paramount in my thoughts before I rang them. Not losing you, but the fact that I had to admit to them that I had failed, in my own terms. I'm sorry for that too.

I haul my heavily empty body out of bed and put on the pale blue quilted dressing gown that I wore that morning in the Lincolnshire garden. It goes round me easily now - almost as well as it did then. My rounded fecundity had been nearly all water. So soon after the delivery, I look as though I have hardly had a baby at all.

The phone is not in its usual place in the hall. Your dad has moved it into the front room, where the fire is, so that I can make my calls in the warmth. I can also sit down on the settee, but for some reason I choose not to. I put the phone on the settee, and sit on the floor in front of it.

I have psyched myself up to make about four phone calls, but then I decide that I can probably get away with two. If I ring one key person on my mum's side of the family, and one on my dad's, they will tell everyone else. I know this will "upset" a lot of people who would want to be told personally, but at the moment I do not give a toss about that and want to make things a little easier for myself.

On my mother's side, I ring the sister that she, and I, were closest to. Many, many times, usually in our kitchen on a winter's evening, my mum would recount the night of my birth, and a key feature of this story was how my dad and Auntie Alice stayed up all night, drinking tea together in the kitchen of my parents' basement flat, waiting for news from the bedroom. It was Auntie Alice who was responsible for my middle name - Lesley. Having no daughters of her own, she pleaded with my mother to adopt this as my middle name almost as soon as I was born, and, as Alice had been there and supported my dad so much, my mum capitulated. It was, as I was to find out as part of my growing up, the way Alice tended to work - she gave kindness, but expected a price to be paid.

As I was growing up, I felt a special bond with Auntie Alice. For, like me, she was very squeamish about any conversation regarding blood, muscles, tendons, ligaments, hamstrings or eyes. While we could manage to look, for instance, at an infected wound, talking about any of these parts of the body would, we used to say, "make our toes turn up." We were the only people we knew who experienced this feeling. It used to make us feel that we shared a special code.

But I have hardly seen Alice since clearing my parents' flat over five years ago, when they had both died. While my dad was still ill in hospital, after my mum had gone, Alice had let me stay at her flat. She had been the one the police had contacted when my mum's body was found, and she had gone to the flat with another of my mother's sisters, Auntie Pauline, to clean up the mess left by my mother on her last night on this earth. I also remember that she has always been the family grapevine - long silences between my mother and her family would be punctuated by Auntie Alice providing news of a birth, impending marriage, or a death.

Yet, despite these moments of remembered contact, the phone call is as bad as I had feared. It is too long since we have spoken. We have forgotten our codes, and cannot re-establish them with news of a dead baby. Auntie Alice likes to be the bringer of good or bad tidings - not to be told them. I know that she will tell the rest of my mother's family very effectively about you, but she cannot find anything to say to me, and it is like listening to someone struggling to learn to read. She simply does not know how to give me comfort from a distance, and I am unable to supply any words to help the conversation flow. I listen to cold silence, and realise Alice's comfort is of the practical variety only. If she were organising the funeral, or even making me cups of tea, she would be able to cope with the news a lot better.

There is one point only at which her voice becomes slightly animated. This surprises me, because it is perhaps the most gruesome part of the conversation.

"The baby's head didn't develop properly," I inform her.

"Was it deformed, then?"

"Yes"

"Poor little mite. Do they know what causes that then?"

"No, not really. They think it might be genetic."

"Oh. Shame."

"Yes." And that was it. The only spontaneous part of the conversation is over. Like a cloud passing in front of the sun, Alice's voice has again become monosyllabic, monotonous and overly Brightonian. By way of ending this piece of communication, I ask her to let other people in the family know the news, and her voice lightens again. As I hear the click of the receiver, something clicks in my head. There is something I know about Auntie Alice, and I don't know why I've only just remembered This, again, is information that my own mother made part of my growing up. About five years before I was born, Alice had her only child - a boy named Ray. Ray was born with slight spina bifida - not incapacitating, but enough to affect his bowel and bladder control. At the time, Alice was told that she was lucky that it wasn't any worse, but they wouldn't give her the odds on it happening again. Alice was not the sort of woman to take risks, and had had no more children - hence, the chance taken to help name her sisters daughter.

My mother always maintained that Alice blamed her husband for the defect. But now I know. Something had stopped me telling Alice that your condition, Louise, is related to spina bifida and hydrocephalus. It is my mother's side of the family that carries the defective gene. Alice and I have far more in common than our squeamishness. We have had deformed babies, and I, with my daughter, have paid the highest price. After a few minutes, I wrap my dressing-gown more tightly round me, retie the belt and ring the other number. The woman known to me when I was young as Auntie Maureen is not actually an aunt at all, but the wife of a nephew of my dad's. I called them Auntie and Uncle when I was little because, not being born until my parents had been married fifteen years, the generation with whom I should have been contemporary had already grown up. By coincidence, I was a bridesmaid at Ray's wedding on the same weekend that I became a godmother for the first time - to Emma Louise, Maureen's third child and only daughter. It was the 30th of July, 1966 - on the day of Ray's wedding, England won the World Cup.

Maureen doesn't know what to say either, but it no longer matters, because all I can do now is give in to incoherent grief. I no longer care about failure. "I lost the baby. I lost the baby." Then I start crying again. I can articulate no other words. I have an impression of a remembered gentle person listening, puzzled. It is about six months since she heard from me, and that was simply to say I was pregnant. Now this. It's not really what you expect on a rainy Saturday morning in Bromley.

As I put the phone down, I realise Maureen can have normal mornings because her daughter, her third child, her Emma Louise, is alive and now seventeen. I have lost contact with her, my god-daughter, my Emma Louise.

I am never to have my planned daughter, Rebecca Louise. My own Louise is dead. I sit on the floor, feeling that I will never have the energy to move again. I rest my head on my arms. The tears that fall onto my sleeve are fractured diamonds. I feel the skin around my eyes puffing, reddening. After a long, long time, I pull something called my body off the floor and go in search of a bath. I do not understand how I will get through the day.

This is my first bath since the delivery. I lock the door. I do not want to be found. I take my pad off very carefully. I am still bleeding, and it seems right that I should be.

In the hot water - about as hot as I can stand it - I lie down. For a while I just look straight ahead at the wallpaper - curious flamingoes on a blue background. We have done no decorating yet. But my eyes cannot help it and I have to look down at my empty, draining body.

I know my dressing gown goes round me easily now, but I am still surprised at how small my tummy looks - a little rounded hill, the dark hair showing quite clearly beyond it. True, I lack muscle tone, but I also lack substance. My hand passes over my skin, beneath the water. There are no stretch marks. I have been left with nothing.

Except my breasts. Their growth unnoticed while my stomach was vast, now they are the most noticeable part of my body. They look hugely overripe, with areolae enlarged enough to accommodate the hungriest baby's mouth. I feel my hand move over the flatness of my stomach, towards the nipple. I almost squeeze, to find out if there is any colostrum. But I stop myself. I do not want to know. I don't want to think about the milk coming in. Perhaps it won't.

After I am dressed, there is a phone call for me. The telephone is back in its customary place in the icy hall. I hear Pam Summerfield's voice.

"I'm so sorry, Penny."

It's the obvious beginning, but Pam, who comes across as a very strong person, says it in a way that suggests this is not empty rhetoric, but that, in some way, she will be able to help. She goes on,

"Jayne told is all on Wednesday, when you were going through it. We carried on but it was all very..."

"Subdued?" I echo the word Jayne used.

"Yes. How are you feeling now?"

"Drained. Confused. Bloody awful. Today, I've had to ring family and tell them. One was my aunt, and that's made me realise that's where the faulty gene came from. And the other was my cousin, who has a seventeen-year-old daughter, that she had after two boys. That brought it home that I haven't just lost a baby, that I didn't just want Louise as a baby - I wanted her as a child, a teenager, I wanted her around as an adult. I've lost her whole life."

"Are you close to your family?"

"No. That's made it worse too. If my mum were still alive, she would have done the informing. She would have acted as some kind of go-between." Suddenly I see, how much I miss my mum - as if I didn't have enough pain already, and I am fighting back yet more tears.

"Yes. I found that telling people was awful when Steve was killed."

"Steve?"

"Heather's father. He was killed in a car crash about a year after Heather was born."

"My God. Pam. I'm so sorry. I always assumed that your husband was her father."

"No. Colin was actually Steve's best friend. It was grieving for him that eventually brought the two of us together."

"I see." There is a silence while I absorb this information. It seems that I have joined a club - the Bereaved Club, in which you are entitled to information about yourself and others, normally concealed from the world. And while the words I say to Pam are no different from those I said to Jayne when she told me about her babies, I say them with authority, for my experience has given me a membership card.

"Pam?"

"Yes?"

"Will the milk come in?"

"Almost certainly, I'm afraid. Especially as you breastfed before." "Oh."

"Well, you know where I am, if it does. And I'm sure Jean Lennox will be able to give you good advice."

"Thanks."

I go out of the way to replace the receiver soundlessly. Then there is a knock. Dr Walker's head appears at the door to the flat.

"Hi. Come in." I can hear the listlessness in my voice as I show him into the front room.

Sam is bouncing around, dancing to a tape. Benjamin is engaged in making a Lego model. Apparently fortified by this display of normal, healthy activity, Dr Walker ventures,

"You don't seem to be as positive as when I saw you the other night."

"No. It's all closing in on me now."

I look at Benjamin as intently as he is studying his Lego plans. I feel that I have failed, or cheated, my doctor along with everyone else. I lulled him into thinking I was fine on Thursday evening. In no way can I think that what I felt there was genuine. This is the truth, this is what it feels like, this is how it is meant to be. Reluctantly, I meet his pale gaze.

"I'm sorry. To tell you the truth, I don't know if I'm coping or not."

"Would you like some homoeopathic stuff to help with the grief?"

"Okay"

He delves into his briefcase and produces white powders for me to take. I cannot actually know if they will make any difference - I don't know what I would have been like anyway.

He is just leaving as Grannie turns up, having made the journey from Birmingham. It's not the journey she hoped to make, at the time she hoped to make it, but she too is someone who can offer practical help, although I know she will not want to dwell on the loss of you. But I am quite prepared for her to do the cooking, cleaning, and whatever it takes to be absolved of the need to care for your brothers. I can still love them, but I cannot do anything for them. I can do nothing for anyone - least of all, myself.

All day it rains, or it is damp outside, with sea mist. The few remaining pink roses in our front garden submit their heads to the leaden winter weather. After lunch, which your grannie gets, I sit in the sprung rocking chair and stare into the middle distance. I have interacted with people nearly all morning. I am exhausted. Then, at about three-thirty, I realise how dark it is getting. We are so near the solstice. I cannot let this day just dissolve into nothing. I have to mark it in some way. I decide to go and see the lights in Kings Road, our local shopping area, which leads down to the sea. Every year, I have been told, the local traders club together to provide Christmas lights. I want to go and see them for the first time, and share them with you.

Whatever inarticulate motive gets me out of the house, I find that it is fulfilled. It lifts me to see people doing their Christmas shopping, the lights holding back the darkness, comforting. I feel that you are here, as much as if I am showing you your first Christmas. But I also realise I want to shop for new underwear. Even if the milk comes in, I don't still have to be wearing the MAVA bras that Tessa ordered through the NCT before I had Sam, that I wore at the end of that pregnancy and right through the eight months that I breastfed him. I have been wearing them for some time now, but they are bras for women with healthy babies. Although, in showing you the Christmas lights, I feel close to you, I know you will also understand that I want to buy ordinary bras, designed to support only my femaleness, not my reproductive capacity. But as I turn a corner, and hear a baby cry, I feel the familiar tingle in my breasts of the first let-down reflex since your birth. My body is ready to feed you. My milk and my love - waiting to give. But the milk, at least, will stop, and instinctively, I know it will be somehow therapeutic to look to a time beyond lactation. There is an old-fashioned corsetry shop near the sea front, and I think that will do perfectly. I want to buy from somewhere cosy, steeped in tradition. I want utilitarian underwear that, as far as possible, has nothing to do with sex.

The bell tings as I go in. There are two glass counters, forming an L-shape, and boxes behind them, stacked up to the ceiling. It all seems a very good sign. Then a man emerges from the back of the shop. I am somewhat taken aback by this, but from his "How can I help you, madam?" I realise that he has had this shop for years, and for some reason, has chosen to specialise in the sale of women's underwear.

I give him the measurements, and explain that I want quite a lot of support from the bras, on account of my childbearing.

"Of course," he says, "any woman who's had children will need it."

"Yes," I agree. "Quite."

We proceed with the purchase, and I choose two white cotton bras with sensibly wide straps. It is as he is wrapping them in white tissue paper, ready to put into their boxes, that he asks,

"How many children have you got?"

I do not know how to reply, and all the possible answers jockey for position at the front of my mind.

"Two."

"Three."

"Three, but one's just died."

I opt for the second. I can't deny your existence, and yet I have to conceal your death, in this shop, talking to a man I do not know.

"Then you should find that this particular make of bra is what you need. How old is your youngest child?"

Again, I hesitate. I suspect he thinks I'm making it up. If I admit how old you really are, he'll wonder why I'm out alone now, without you. I know I can't pretend that Sam is my youngest child - my figure is all wrong for it.

"I had a child a few days ago, but she died." I have said it. My heart is thumping, my face is flushed. I am cornered, but I have said it.

"Oh my dear," he says, "I'm so sorry. Let me open the door for you."

I have gathered my purchases together, and am able to leave the shop with some dignity. I know that I can do this now - to complete strangers, I can admit this dreadful tragedy. It will never be so hard again.

And then, as the seadamp, nightdark air hits my face and ears and nostrils, I wonder again why it should be me facing this, trying to learn to be brave, to handle the reaction of other people as well as my own grief. I know life isn't fair, but why me?

Turning back into Kings Road, the Christmas lights now only mock the futility of the idea that anything can be done to dismiss the dark, to send it back, to pretend that we can, in any way, lighten our darkness or our burdens. You are no longer with me as I walk back, and I don't know where you are when I cannot feel you here. I am a piece of brackish seaweed, washed up at high tide on the bitter shingle, at the mercy of forces I cannot begin to comprehend.

33 Heavenly Peace

Round yon virgin mother and child
Holy infant so tender and mild
Sleep in heavenly peace
Sleep in heavenly peace

The following day, I'm not quite sure what persuades me to take your grannie to the St. Andrew's Carol Service, as the light fails for the fourth time since your birth. I haven't spent the day anticipating going, or even consciously aware that it is to take place. And apart from your service in the chapel on Thursday, it is years since I have set foot in a religious building. The nearest I come these days is our weekly jaunt up the hill to toddler group.

I think, partly, we go because, at twilight, the same restlessness comes over me as I felt the day before, when I took you to see the lights. I have spent the day keeping quietly still, for two interrelated reasons - one physical, one, emotional. The let-down reflex of the day before did indeed herald things to come, and the milk has come in. Sod's Law dictates that, while I struggled to produce enough milk for your brothers, now, it is gushing out, painfully. Some instinct has told me that it will be better if I keep still, contained within myself. This is totally congruent with the other idea I have that, if I move too fast, the hurt contained within me will cascade out, like the milk, from an anguish too great to be borne. I have rung Pam, whose advice is to wear tight bras and try not to remove them until the flow has ceased. I am grateful for my new underwear, even if it was purchased at some emotional expense. I wear one of the bras on its tightest fastening and add hankies for extra pressure. My breasts are more comfortable now, but I am dreading having to take my bra off the following day when I have my bath.

Emotionally, as night falls, I feel no different, but I need to redeem the day - not to let it pass unmarked, with only the pain, or its avoidance, remembered. The Carol Service, with its spiritual element, lightening the darkness, seems as good a way as any of doing this, and it is accessible.

I know your grannie will go happily because she is a church-going person anyway. She has a faith. I do not want to take your brothers. I know it will be a family occasion but I still need uninterrupted time. Your dad is willing to have them again. The sense of spiritual appropriateness has not settled on him in the same way.

As we leave the house, I feel the coldness of the coming night on my face, and take a sharp intake of breath. I am so afraid of cold - of real winter weather. Since the cloud passed over the sun on Tuesday, on my way from the university, the weather has been dark and damp – cotton-wool weather and for that, at least, I can be grateful. Weather that called me to see winter's fractured colours or feel cold in stabbing clarity would splinter my glass shell into jagged refractive shards. And for a moment, I fear the weather is changing, moving towards this. But it is only the coming of night, and there are no stars to stab me, only low, amorphous clouds.

Our road, Chapel Park Road, rises steeply towards the top, as I can testify from my many walks that way. They have become increasingly difficult these last months, but now, there is nothing in my uterus to prevent me ever doing anything at all. St. Andrew's Church, a dark brick cube, stands imposingly on the hill. It is a characteristically Anglo-Catholic church, built towards the end of the last century, where it could self-consciously be seen to be fulfilling both its spiritual and social missions.

Inside, with soft lighting, partly from the flames of many, many candles, we can see the drill redness of the brick in the pillars flanking the nave. Already we seem warmer. Although we are early, the church is packed with families, with children, with people apparently at ease. Your grannie and I find a pew near the back. We are not in the central aisle, and it is slightly darker here. We will not be able to see so much; there will be people in the way of what is happening; I don't mind. I welcome the feeling of darkness on my face.

Above the heads of the people, unknown but unthreatening, I can see Michael's shawl-coloured hair. It seems lighter and his fringe seems to have a bounce to it - perhaps he has washed it. This is only the second time I have seen him in his vestments - the second time in three days...

Keeping my emotions in check, I look again at Michael, the altar he stands in front of, the huge stained glass window behind him, and up, up and around the church, taking in its impressive space and vaulted height. Three days ago, he stood as he stands now, before an altar, but in a tiny chapel, framed by an exquisite stained glass window. That, he did for you, the child born to death, beyond consciousness. And whatever meaning I can give to God was there. It was with Michael, it was with you, it was with the handful of people who were there. Now he stands before hundreds of people to celebrate a coming child, a living child - and yet, as on Thursday, there is no child. There is only what we choose to make conscious, what we believe.

I hold myself together until the carols come, so redolent of my own childhood – especially "Away in a Manger." Michael has reserved the first verse for the children to sing. It suddenly hits me that you will never sing them, or be in a school play or nativity, playing Mary (something I was never asked to do) or a shepherd or a king with a tea towel wrapped around your head, for there is no head around which to secure it. You are dead to any meaning we can assign to religious festivals, and their trappings and culture as well. I cry without sound, and only your grannie notices. She looks at me quickly then looks away without speaking. I simply let my tears fall onto the somewhat battered and now unfamiliar coat that I can now get into. I could go on doing this, I think - sobbing in darkened spaces, surrounded by an unaware public - but my nose gives me away. Its contents dribble onto my top lip, and I have to sniff loudly, cutting the atmosphere. Your grannie passes me a hanky. I blow my nose, and by that decisive act I am able to cease crying and lock my pain, temporarily, in another part of my being.

In the sermon, Michael says something about how Mary must have felt coming to the end of the pregnancy - at long last the baby was nearly due, but she had the trauma of a long journey on a donkey, then the labour, before she could welcome her son into the world. All of a sudden, I am insanely jealous of Mary, who was allowed to keep her baby, and give birth to him, living, at this time of the year. It doesn't make the slightest difference that I have had two living baby sons. If Mary was allowed to keep her son, why wasn't I allowed to keep my daughter? Because he was God's son too, and God gets to make the decisions. It simply is not fair, it's not fair, what right does God have to decide these things for us? I know that, in time to come, I will relate infinitely more closely to the poignancy of the *Stabat Mater* image than ever before, but for now, I want to gouge Mary's eyes out because her son was thirty-three before he died. Strangely enough, this fierce negativity gives me a focus for the service, and I throw myself into what remains of it, even greeting the few people I know at the end, and introducing them to my mother-in-law.

We go home to a family tea which your brothers have helped your dad to make. It's a traditional English tea of sandwiches, salad and cakes, all laid out on our old-fashioned wooden table, which lives in the bay window of the front room. It comforts me to remember how much it resembles the one my parents had for years. We are to choose what we want and eat away from the table - adults on comfortable chairs, your brothers on the floor. We use the reindeer mugs, and they are simply the reindeer mugs, devoid of symbolism. I love my family.

The doorbell rings. I walk through the lighted hall and open the big front door. It is Alison and Michael. He is dressed in his deep black cloak, a winter night's costume unchanged through centuries. I can see only his head, and his cheeks and hair and sharp jaw are the colour of bone in the harsh light. He has come on an errand of destiny. Alison is wearing her duffle coat.

They claim that they thought they saw me at the concert, so they decided to come and see how I was. I ask them in warily. Apart from my murderous thoughts towards Mary, which I do not think will impress Michael overmuch, one carol service does not make a convert, and I suspect they may now think I am ready to join their club. I want something from this club, I want it to be there for me, especially at the moment, but I also want to preserve a spiritual freedom and not to be circumscribed by an organised religion. Also, there are too many confused thoughts already in my head for me to be able to take any kind of consistent intellectual stand, if they want to argue it out. But I decide that, perhaps after all, tea can be just tea, and I have reinforcements in the shape of adults and children if I need them.

They are welcomed into the room and invited to partake of the food on offer. Benjamin and Sam help them in their choices, while your grannie makes fresh tea. When they are ensconced with their rations, the conversation splinters. Alison and I start a women's chat, while your dad and Michael go into a blokey huddle, and your grannie deals with the needs of your brothers. It's the first time I have had a chance to speak to Alison alone since our meeting that afternoon in November, when I was someone else. Effortlessly, she provides the next instalment in the story.

"I've finished all those tablets now, that cost us so much, so we're trying again. Nothing's happened yet, but I'm so fed up of waiting. So I've told my uterus, 'You will get pregnant this month.'" She looks down at her abdomen. I dismiss this possibility. Experience of friends has told me that people who consciously think of becoming pregnant often don't. I have some kind of idea how devastatingly hurt I would be if Alison were to become pregnant at this time, but because Alison is my friend, I put this from me too. Even if there were some kind of retribution at work for my earlier insensitivity, I would not deserve this.

34 A Viewing and a Funeral

Wonder if you understand
It's just the touch of your hand
Behind a closed door
All I needed was the love you gave
All I needed for another day
And all I ever knew
Only you

It is the next day - Monday. Exactly one week since the Meet-a-Mum party and my meeting with Sister Neep, in which I admitted to her how long I had wanted you for, and to myself, how close I was to holding you for always. Now, today is the last chance any of us will ever have to see you. Tomorrow you will be buried. For today, you are at rest in the funeral director's. It is five days to Christmas. Your grannie wants to see you, and your dad will take her this afternoon. I will stay here at the flat and look after your brothers. Nothing is left for me in being only with your body. I have said my goodbyes.

Late in the morning, I go for my bath. Removing my bra, which I do as the water is running, is every bit as bad as I had feared. A searing, scarlet, tingly pain floods into my breasts as l suspend them pendulously above the bath and involuntarily allow the milk to flow. There is a flood which diminishes to a steady trickle, then a drip, then nothing. I get into my ridiculously nutritious bath. After I have finished, I watch the whitened liquid drain away. This wastage hurts, in every way possible.

After lunch, Sister Lennox arrives to check me. Back on her own rounds, visiting patients in their own homes, she has regained the confidence missing when she visited me in the Dexter. She is the caring, competent nurse I remember, with a rounded figure and honest amber eyes, and her hat sits neatly on her head. She examines me thoroughly. It has been an amazingly clean delivery. She checks my pad, and that is fine. There is no sign of clotting, or haemorrhage. Her hands examine my abdomen. Even without the advantages of breastfeeding, my uterus has already returned to its normal size and correct position, although I still have some work to do on my pelvic floor. Again, more signs that my body is so much more prepared than all the rest of me to forget I had you. I ask about the milk.

"Pam Summerfield suggested wearing really tight bras, and that works at the time, but I have to take them off sometime, and then it kills."

"You could try Epsom Salts. They're an old-fashioned remedy from the days when lots of women lost babies."

"Okay. At the moment, I'll try anything. I wanted to ask some more advice, actually. Paul and I thought of taking the boys to Birmingham for Christmas. After all, there's nothing to celebrate here now, and I think it would be good for us to be with some kind of extended family. Will I be okay to travel?"

"Yes, you'll be fine," she smiled. "Good idea."

I give the Epsom Salts a try, and although they make me retch badly, they do the trick. By the time we leave for Birmingham two days later, the milk has dried up. I do not lament the passing of the physical pain. It's another sign that my body will let you go, but I cannot see it as any kind of healing process. When your dad and grannie return from the funeral director's, all she says is that she is glad she went. She quietly goes to spend time with her living grandchildren, who have missed her. Your dad volunteers more information.

"How did Louise look?" I ask. I know there is no mileage in the question for me, but feel the need to ask it anyway.

"Different."

"How different?"

"Well - they'd put something on her face, to give her some colour - a nice pink. But there was nothing to support her head, like there was at the hospital, when she had so many blankets round it. It was still covered, but you could see how flat it was, how bad it was. But she looked so pretty. She'd have been a lovely girl."

He weeps soundlessly, and we hold each other, while I try to visualise what they have done - accentuated your abnormality while turning you into a doll. Once the image is crystallised, I hold it at the front of my head as tenaciously as I hold your dad in my arms. I must hold on to what is, not speculate on what might have been. That is its own huge sea of pain, into which I have dipped a toe but as yet, I am ready to go no further, for I will soon be out of my depth.

Lesley phones in the evening and asks if I would like her to come to the funeral. I say yes.

It is now exactly a week since we saw a sunny day, and, for your funeral, it is raining. You are to be buried in the morning. There will be no ceremony beforehand - it is simply that we will be there before you are put into the ground. Your brothers are to go to Tina's, because we simply don't think they are old enough to understand, and young child behaviour is not what we want to cope with there. It is not that we don't want to involve them, or we have a misplaced idea that we are shielding them from something.

We travel in two cars. Your dad takes your grannie, Michael and Lesley, and I go with Alison and Rosie. I notice a crucifix attached to the steering wheel of Alison's car, and it makes me feel somewhat uneasy.

We have a long way to walk, once we reach the cemetery. Michael leads the way, for he knows where you are to be buried. I look around, and in this rain I can pick out no landmarks or reference points. I will never be able to find my way here again, without help. Your resting place will also be lost to me, but somehow this does not matter, for I know that your body is not where your soul will be: I know that I will never again find you here. The wet pebbles of the tortuous pathways shine and crunch beneath our feet. Then we branch off and take a muddy walk between obscure graves. We are now at the very edge of the cemetery. We are where only the unknown and unnamed are buried. We are here at the right time, only just ahead of the funeral directors, who are approaching with a white box, which seems not much bigger than a shoe box. I could never have imagined that even your newborn and undeveloped body could fit in something so tiny. As the men lift you off their shoulders I can see the inscription on the lid of the coffin.

Baby Sutherland
At rest

For a fraction of a second, I feel outraged that the fact you were stillborn deprives you of a name. And then my chest opens and I relax: this is right. For Baby Sutherland, even with all that your dad and I invested in her, is your body only, and it is truly over. It is Louise who lives on in our hearts, minds and corners of our beings. It is Louise with whom we will still have some kind of relationship. If the name calls you into being, Louise is your soul.

The rain has now changed to a drizzle driven by the wind. Your dad and I hold each other as Michael says a few words, and the funeral directors carry on around him: if we were not here, there would be nothing. Many stillborn babies lie here; without blessing, and I think of them too, beside you.

There is another space next to yours; they are saving one for later. Your dad and I continue to cling to each other as your tiny white box is lowered into the ground, and I smell the wet fabric of his Hornes overcoat against my cheek. We cry together for all we have lost, and I want to stay in the moment forever, but your grannie decides that we have had enough.

"Come on," she insists. "Leave her now. Let's go back to Benjamin and Sam."

Slowly, your dad and I release our hold of each other. This is the third time we said goodbye to you, and the last. I go round hugging all the other people who have come to say goodbye to you and support us. I look into eyes as deep in sorrow as my own. My own grief melds with theirs. We all walk back to the cars in silence, the drizzle meeting our faces.

Everyone who has been at the graveside comes back to the flat for some tea and sandwiches. Many of these people have never met before, yet there is a friendly, relaxed atmosphere, as they swap personal details. I overhear Lesley telling Rosie that she has three daughters, and it hurts that I cannot use that word in relation to myself. Sharon Clayton turns up, her long hair tied back again, droplets of mist on the curls framing her fine forehead. She tells me she has left something for me in the kitchen which she wants me to open only when I have a private moment.

It is raining the following day too when we stack the Avenger with the presents we had expected to open in St. Leonards, and set off for Birmingham.

References

Like you, Louise, most of the songs, poems and books I've quoted from are those closest to my heart. There is much here that I would have wanted to share in your life, but can do it only through this book. I did not go and look for the quotations as I was writing - mostly, they came and found me; either remembered phrases that came into my head, or texts I was reading that I understood would inform what I was trying to say.

Being now intertwined with the part of my being that is you, they are now changed for me forever.

Chs. 1-18 Donovan *Legend of a Girl Child Linda* from *Sunshine Superman*.

During most of 1970 I studied English at Hendon College of Technology - unlikely but true. I used to listen to a friend's copy of the album - often through the residence walls - in a desultory sort of way, but often found myself writing poetry that echoed the images in this song. I rediscovered it at another friend's house in 1976 and recorded it. It was there for you when needed

Chs. 3&4 TS Eliot *Journey of the Magi*

I first discovered Eliot when I started in the sixth form, and was introduced to his work by an American student teacher. She took us through The Love Song of J Alfred Prufrock at the same time. While the profundity of the work moved me, I felt able to relate to much of it. The Prufrock lines in particular are repeated in the book, as they were often repeated through my life. Since you, they have had little relevance. I do not expect my dreams to be realised. I expect only to make the best of what I have.

Ch. 4 TS Eliot *Burnt Norton* from *The Four Quartets*.

This book had a profound effect on me when I studied Eliot for an Artist and Public in Contemporary Society course at Sussex. While there was a lot I didn't understand, the synergy of words, metre and meaning created for me something so momentous I could only wonder.

Ch. 9 TS Eliot *Marina*

This was another poem I discovered on the same course. The image of the ship, which is in my blood, my daughter, the dreams and their tearing- they all prefigure On Living Water.

Ch. 10 back to *Burnt Norton*

Ch. 11 Edward Thomas *October*

Thomas' poetry was one of the texts I had to study at 'A' level. I found him an enigmatic poet and difficult to write about. Now, although I think I would have the same trouble putting pen to paper, it is precisely that elusiveness that I appreciate. The other reference is Burnt Norton again. This would have been the point at which my life had set, if not for you.

Ch. 13 Kahlil Gibran *The Prophet*

Rosie James actually introduced me to this while I was pregnant with you. I already understood these words in my head. Now I know their validity in the marrow.

Ch. 15 TS Eliot *Little Gidding*

My favourite, and the most perfect of the Quartets. If only there were another way of bringing it to you.

Ch. 16 *The Prophet* again.

I own the consequences of my actions

Ch. 17 *Prufrock* see ch.4

Ch. 19 Virginia Woolf *A Writer's Diary*

Mrs Dalloway was another of my A Level texts. I have had a fairly close relationship with Virginia Woolf since, not least because she drowned herself at Rodmell, Sussex. I would have wanted to offer you an appreciation of her life and work as a feminist writer.

Ch. 20 also *Burnt Norton* again.

I hope you are happy with the juxtaposition of Virginia Woolf and TS Eliot. Their politics may have been far apart, but there are many parallels to be made in their work. One day, I would like to explore this further.

Chs. 21&22 *East Coker* The second of the *Quartets*.

My Auntie Midge used to live in the next village to East Coker, and I did the pilgrimage in the summer of 1977. It was very hot, as opposed to Little Gidding, which I visited with your dad one very cold winter's Sunday afternoon - appropriately. But the church was dosed.

Ch. 23 Richard Harris *Macarthur Park*

I fell deeply in love for the first time with one of the painters who came to paint the outside of our school shortly before my seventeenth birthday. For me, it was a blissful few weeks and by the time I realised he wasn't going to come back for me, I was already starting to get over it. This song, which came out that summer, was always associated with him, and, for me, the poignancy of that first green and eager love that never really comes again. That's still there, but of course, it is now overlaid with knowing of the unanswered question which is you.

Ch. 24 The Flying Pickets *Only You*

I still hope to avoid hearing this song by accident. I have to prepare myself for It. I just hear those opening bars, and all that you meant, and mean, floods back to me - every loss, every gain.

Prufrock The last and most desperate reference. see chs.4 & 17

Ch. 25 *Only You* again

Chs 26,27,28 *Little Gidding*. Oh God

Ch. 29 *Only You*

Ch. 30 *Burnt Norton*

Ch. 31 *Only You*

Ch. 32 *Burnt Norton*

Ch. 33 *Silent Night*
You are the purity of this, and all carols associated with children.

Ch. 34 *Only You*